Medicine in the
Stranglehold of Profit

Thomas Hardtmuth, MD

Medicine
in the stranglehold
of profit

**The threat to the art of healing and the
social fabric – and the new orientation needed
for truly looking after health**

With an afterword by Richard House, PhD

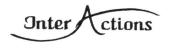

First published in German as
*Medizin in Würgegriff des Profits –
Die Gefährdung der Heilkunst
durch die Gesetze der Ökonomie*
AmThor Verlag 2017

Translation by
Richard Brinton

English edition with additional Afterword
Published in the UK by
InterActions 2023

www.interactions360.org
contact@interactions360.org

ISBN 978-1-915594-00-6

Cover illustration by Felix Hardtmuth
Printed in the UK

Contents

Preface to the English Edition

This text is a revised and expanded version of a lecture given on 11.5.2017 at Café Walden, Talhof Heidenheim.

The occasion was the increasingly precarious financial situation of the local hospital, where the author worked as a surgeon for over 25 years. At most municipal hospitals, the medical and nursing care mandate is increasingly being distorted by an economic logic of competition and growth, as is common in industrial companies. The takeover of hospitals by hospital groups further intensifies this pressure and ultimately endangers the culture of medical care. The intention of the lecture was to make a contribution to the preservation of the clinic in municipal sponsorship and to clarify the actual, financial-market-political backgrounds that are hidden behind the bogus concept of the cost explosion in the health care system.

This English edition is coming out six years after the original, but what is described in the book – the very deep problems coming from a profit-driven business model for health care – is more relevant than ever. When health care becomes a business, with for instance priority given to profits for shareholders, actual health considerations will inevitably suffer. As I demonstrate in the text that follows, over the past half century the 'health care industry' has increasingly moved into underhand tactics, fraud and corruption in order to maximise their gains. By 2017 the pharmaceutical industry, for instance, had the worst reputation of all business sectors.

The business strategies used for profit and gain within the health care industry have not changed in recent years since the 2017 German edition of this book; they have only multiplied further and if anything have become more refined. My presentation doesn't just dwell, though, on the pitfalls inherent in the current trends and its ill effects on society but considers what is needed for health care to become truly health oriented, with then its positive effects on the well-being of society. Richard House takes up these aspects further in his Afterword.

Introduction

Let us introduce this evening's topic with two quotes; the first is from Harald Lesch, professor of astrophysics in Munich and presenter of well-known scientific television programs. In one of these broadcasts he asked himself the question, why are so many crimes committed? His answer: because of money.

'Some crimes are committed so that the perpetrator can get the money that the person who was killed had. But you could also get money more easily. You don't have to kill someone to get it. You could get money by committing completely different crimes. Between you and me, I think large parts of the international financial world are criminal. I think what is happening is a crime. It is not only an offence against morality, but it is an offence against everything we hold high and sacred, at least in this part of the world. The fact that a few are enriching themselves at the expense of the general public, enriching themselves so much that they no longer know what to do with all the money, I consider that a capital crime. You are welcome to google what capital crime means in German. In this case it really is a crime with capital and for capital and because of capital. That's what I consider to be the perfect crime, on the face of it. What has happened in the last decades is perfection in its purest form. Structures that have been built up and do nothing but multiply money, and this money then looks for investments to multiply further. In the meantime, trillions are traded in a virtual market that no one controls any more. Computers trade with computers, money is created out of nothing, although we always know that nothing comes from nothing.' (Friedrich & Weik, 2014)

This painting by the German painter Sascha Schneider from 1896 shows Mammon and his slave. Mammon represents the rule of money, the empire of the market, to whose laws we have subjected ourselves – this market, becomes an anonymous master without a face, who here assumes a quasi-religious status with his halo. Even his slave cannot show his face.

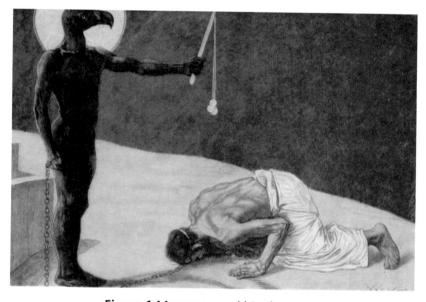

Figure 1 Mammon and his slave

The second quote comes from Giovanni Maio; he is an internist and philosopher and is a professor of medical ethics at the University of Freiburg. He is one of the most prominent and eloquent campaigners against the increasing economisation of medicine. He has published his thoughts on this subject in the book *Geschäftsmodell Gesundheit – wie der Markt die Heilkunst abschafft* [*Business Model Health – How the Market is Abolishing the Art of Healing*], which is well worth reading (Maio, 2014).

The inappropriate transfer of economic rationality to medicine cannot go well in the long run. Not even the hoped-for reduction in costs has occurred. Instead, there has been an increase in lucrative interventions, yet often with questionable implications. Even more serious is the gradual distortion of the logic of medical care. Nowadays doctors are implicitly taught to classify patients in economic categories and to reflect on the balance sheet of each patient. Chronically ill patients, patients with many illnesses, patients with a risk of complications, patients with a high cost of care all promise a bad balance sheet. One tends to try to avoid such patients because they fall off the efficiency grid. The social question of how to help people is replaced by the strategic question of where help is still profitable. The more uncertain the result, the greater the pressure to justify taking care of the person in need. If the business interest overrides the need of the person concerned to such an extent that the sick person is not seen as a call for help but as a threat to the balance sheets, then this leads to an alienation of the helping professions from their own identity and thus plunges them into a crisis of meaning in their actions. This crisis of meaning is intensified by the fact that a new culture of dealing with the patient is also being established under economic domination. Doctors still deliver high technical quality, but they save on contact time with the patient. Because the economised operation is completely synchronised, no time is reserved for anything outside the predefined cycle. In this way, a bustle is established that makes it virtually impossible for doctors to react spontaneously to patients and to really respond to them. The result is the introduction of a structurally conditioned depersonalisation between doctor and patient. It is not the conscientious doctor who takes time and is personally involved who is rewarded but the doctor who makes quick decisions without spending a lot of time and material. Many doctors, however, then feel that they did not qualify for such a form of medicine when they visited the lecture halls. It is becoming increasingly clear that if medicine only follows economic logic it will no longer be medicine in the end. Therefore, medicine must reflect on its basic social identity and advocate for such an implementation of economic thinking that enables it to remain what it must be from the patients' point of view: a discipline of authentic care for the whole person.[1]

So this book is not about a general criticism of economic thinking in medicine but about an appropriate balance between economics and medicine, and I would like to try to show where this balance becomes skewed. I will try to show why more and more hospitals are going bankrupt or at least in the red, as is the case here in Heidenheim, although this hospital performs very well at a very high level.

---

1   This particular Giovanni Maio quote is from the journal *Forschung und Lehre*, April 2013.

The global financial market

To understand today's situation in the health sector we need to take a brief historical look back at the development of the global financial market since the 1970s. Before 1971, the financial market was largely under national control and relatively manageable; someone was responsible for every capital transaction, so to speak. Now, in 1971, something happened that many economists believe marked the beginning of global madness: on 15 August 1971, the then USA President Richard Nixon removed the dollar's gold peg. Until then, the Bretton Woods Agreement applied, according to which only as many dollars could be spent as were deposited as the corresponding gold value. As a result of the Vietnam War, the USA had put so many dollars into circulation, or 'squandered' them in the truest sense of the word, that the corresponding gold reserves were no longer sufficient. In 1973, the Bretton Woods Agreement was completely abolished, all exchange rates were liberalised and capital controls were largely removed. This was the beginning of the deregulation of the financial markets.

Now keep this event in mind for our further considerations. On the following charts I have marked this point in time with a red arrow, which will now appear again and again. In the following years the complete deregulation of the financial markets or stock exchange trading was pushed further and further, in which Margaret Thatcher in London also played a major role. 'Let's throw away all the rules that slow down success' was the motto. This development was also further accelerated in Germany. First, in 1991, the Kohl government abolished the stock exchange turnover tax and replaced it with the Financial Market Promotion Act [Finanzmarktförderungsgesetz]; in 1997 the wealth tax was abolished, and in the following years the value-added tax was increased three times. Under the Schröder government corporate tax was virtually halved, and the top tax rate was gradually reduced from 53 to 42 and then to 33.7 % today. The tax rate for the super-rich, i.e. people who own more than €174 million, was cut from 43.6% to 23.7%. All these tax giveaways for the wealthy or for the financial sector naturally tore big holes in the federal budget. The last act in the deregulation of the financial markets took place on November 12, 1999 by the government under Bill Clinton in the U.S. where a law was repealed which had been worked out in 1933 by the then senators Carter Glass and Henry B. Steagall (Glass Steagall Act). This act contained the strict separation of commercial and investment banks. This was intended to prevent another global economic depression like the one in the 1920s. The new law (Gramm-Leach-Bliley Act) now enabled speculators and investment bankers not only to gamble with their own money, but they suddenly had access to the money of savers, insured persons and pensioners.

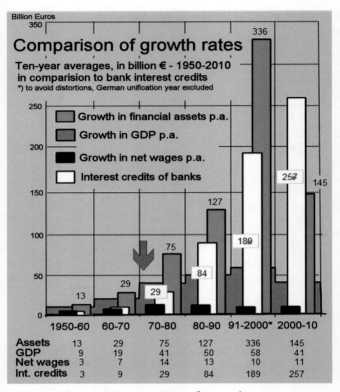

Figure 2 Comparison of growth rates

The liberalisation of the financial markets was linked to two factors that set something in motion worldwide that can be called a social carcinoma; a carcinoma is something that detaches itself from the context of the whole and develops an independent, proliferating life of its own in the organism and destroys it over time. This cancerous growth in the social organism is called the global financial market. The term financial product should actually be chosen as the word of the year, because behind this term there is no value creation in the sense of a product but basically a parasitic entity.

A concrete example may illustrate this: After the financial bubble burst in 2008, speculators discovered raw materials and foodstuffs on the world market as an object of speculation, which led to the world market prices for rice, maize and grain rising within a short time, in some cases by several hundred percent. This in turn had the consequence that millions of people were driven to the abyss of starvation. At the time, the presenter of the *Heute* Journal, Claus Kleber, was filming a documentary on the causes of global hunger and found out that in India heaps of grain bags the size of a football pitch were rotting, serving as a speculative commodity and, in a sense, being held back from the market in order to keep prices high. Just a few hundred metres away people lived in hunger and misery in the slums. In India, about 1 million children die of starvation every year due to malnutrition – one sixth of this rotten speculative commodity would have been enough to prevent this.

Let us now return to the two factors that have further exacerbated the global imbalance in the social fabric. The unpegging of the dollar from gold has now caused the banks' capital cover to fall further and further; it is now between 2 and 3% on average. So if you go to the bank today and borrow €10,000 to buy a car, it is enough if the bank has deposited €200 to €300 of its own capital, the rest of this loan is a money creation out of thin air. But if you then buy a car with this money, then this car belongs to the bank until you have paid off the loan. The money that you pay back to the bank, including the interest, comes from a value creation process; it is actually earned money, in contrast to the money creation of the bank. This circumstance has now contributed to the fact that debt has increased dramatically worldwide; the banks were able to lend money without limit, as it were, which they did not actually possess. The second factor that led to the excessive accumulation of capital in fewer and fewer hands worldwide was the fact that income tax was always higher than capital gains tax; in simple words: having money is more profitable than working. This, too, led to an exponential development of wealth, which has resulted in this ever-diverging relationship between rich and poor worldwide to this day. The ten richest people in Germany alone have a fortune of 150 billion Euros. The top eight men in the global ranking have a combined fortune of 426 billion US dollars. That is more than the entire poorer half of the world's population owns – more than three and a half billion people. The fact that fewer and fewer people own more and more is now accepted with astonishing tolerance. If there were real public knowledge and transparency of the situation, a revolution would inevitably break out immediately.

Figure 2 is taken from a monthly report of the Bundesbank and shows a comparison of the growth rates of finances since 1950. You can see the black bars at the bottom, which represent the development of net wages. As is well known, these have not had any significant real growth in the last 40 years. The grey bars represent the growth in gross domestic product, i.e. the amount of total national wealth generated. Already here one can see that net wages have clearly lagged behind the general growth. Wealth has grown accordingly, which can be seen from the increasingly steep rise in the red bars. Here, however, the financial crisis of 2008 is the reason that wealth in Germany was more than halved at that time.

What nevertheless continues to show exponential growth is the investment income or interest credits of the banks. There we have an extremely disproportionate increase over the last 50 years. Note our red arrow, which marks the beginning of the deregulation of the financial markets. This period now also marks the beginning of the rapid increase in government debt.

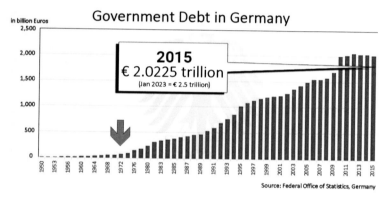

Figure 3 Government debt in Germany

This chart shows the development of public debt in Germany over the last 50 years. We now have a debt level of over 2 trillion Euros. In 2010, the interest burden on public budgets was 61.5 billion Euros, which is almost the entire hospital budget in Germany.

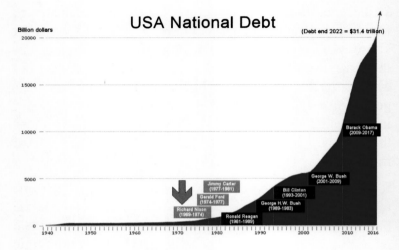

Figure 4 USA national debt

The next chart shows the development of public debt in the USA since 1940; here, too, our red arrow marks the rapid rise of this curve. If we were to plot the global debt of the individual countries here, the curve would take an even steeper upward course; the emerging countries in particular are now so massively indebted that they are sinking into an almost complete economic impotence and dependency. In 2016, global debt increased by 7.6 trillion to a total of 215 trillion US dollars. The question now arises, to whom do we actually owe these immense debts? The economists Marc Friedrich and Matthias Weik, authors of the well-known book *The Greatest Robbery in History*[2] (Friedrich & Weik,

2   Marc Friedrich and Matthias Weik, *Der größte Raubzug der Geschichte: Warum die Fleißigen immer ärmer und die Reichen immer reicher werden* ['The greatest robbery in history: Why the hard-working are getting poorer and the rich are getting richer'], Lübbe, 7th edition, 2014

2014), took the liberty of calling the Federal Ministry of Finance [Bundesfinanzministerium] and asking; they didn't know exactly, they were told, but they should try the Bundesbank. There they were told that it was a rather complicated structure! The creditors were those who owned the government bonds and there was a complicated network of investment banks, hedge funds and private individuals. But these things are subject to banking secrecy and no precise information can be given.

It is a widespread psychological tool of deception that one makes unpleasant truths that one does not want to be in the public eye appear so complicated that the normal person no longer understands them. Camouflage through academic complexity, you could call it. But if you work your way through the thicket of capital interconnections, you will find that in the end only a very few remain who have grotesquely high financial assets at their disposal. We must always remember that the debts of some are the assets of others. And as the debts have grown, so have the assets, and this has led to an extreme imbalance in the global distribution of wealth.

The fairy tale of the cost explosion in the healthcare system

Now, in 1974, the term cost explosion in health care suddenly appeared. This explosion metaphor suggested a notion that we were sitting on a ticking time bomb, so to speak, and that the situation was threatening to get out of control. This ticking time bomb would require immediate action and in view of the imminent danger, time-consuming concerns would have to be put aside. Doctors and patients in particular were made to feel guilty with the accusation of wasting money. Numerous economists, however, have critically examined this hypothesis of cost explosion in the health system. It has now become apparent that this concept does not reflect the actual facts at all.

If we look at the development of health care spending in Germany since 1992, we see a significant increase to 344 billion Euros in 2015, but if we compare these costs to the gross domestic product, i.e., to the total economic return, we see that the share of health care costs in the gross domestic product is actually largely stable. Since 1996, it has hovered around 10.5%. The sudden increase in 2008 was due to the financial crisis, in which the gross domestic product went down by more than 5% and thus the relative share of healthcare costs went up in percentage terms (see Figure 5).

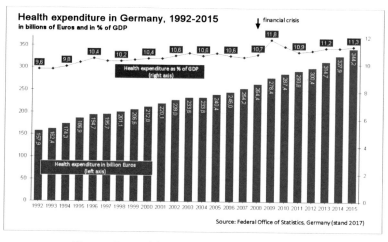

Figure 5 Health expenditure in Germany

So if we look at the development of healthcare costs against the background of the normal consumer price index, we see that in relation to the price development of other areas such as transport, leisure, food, etc., healthcare costs do not differ significantly.

What does show a significant increase, however, is the average contribution rate to statutory health insurance as a percentage of gross wages (see Figure 6). Note again our red arrow; until the 1970s, the contribution to statutory health insurance was always around 8% of gross wages. Since the beginning of the seventies this contribution suddenly increased and today we are at 15.7%.

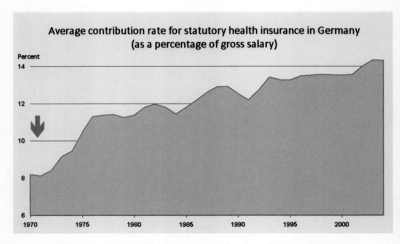

Figure 6 Contribution rates for health insurance

Health expenditure has therefore not risen disproportionately in relation to gross domestic product. What lagged behind the development of the general national wealth, however, were gross wages. We already mentioned that price-adjusted net wages have not increased significantly over the last 40 years (brown curve, Figure 7). So wages have not really participated in the general economic growth – another factor in the widening gap between rich and poor. So if gross wages increase less than gross domestic product, the logical consequence is that the contribution rate to health insurance must increase as a percentage of gross wages.

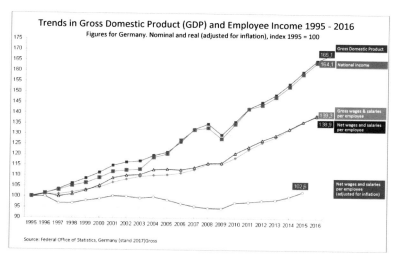

Figure 7 Trends in employee income and GDP

Health reforms have been pushed through in Germany since the mid-seventies with the bogus argument of exploding costs. It began in 1976 with the first cost-cutting measures; here the contributions of the pension fund to the health insurance of pensioners were reduced from 17 to 11 %. In the following years, co-payments were made for medicines, remedies, for massages, spectacles, baths and much more. In 1983, for the first time, patients had to pay an additional DM 5 per day for hospital treatment, which is now 10 Euros. From 1989 onwards, negative lists were drawn up, whereby certain therapeutics such as phyto- and homeotherapeutics were no longer reimbursed. Or fixed amounts were charged for medicines, whereby patients had to pay the difference. GPs were also subject to increasing budgeting; they received only limited reimbursement for hospital admissions, prescriptions, home visits, prescriptions for physiotherapy and much more, i.e. if a GP had issued more than, for example, 100 prescriptions for physiotherapy, he or she was no longer reimbursed for each additional prescription. The list of cuts in the benefits of the statutory health insurance funds now continues with cuts in taxi fares, dentures, cures, practice fees, death benefits and much more. In some cases, the bureaucratic hurdles and the applications for reimbursement of benefits have become so complicated that an amount of about 2 billion Euros has now accumulated due to the non-utilisation of entitled benefits.

Hospitals have not been spared from the cost-cutting measures either. Normally, a hospital has an investment requirement of around 8% of its annual turnover for renovations, maintenance, new acquisitions, etc.; this has been halved to 4% since the 1990s. In addition, rising costs due to tariff increases, growing energy costs and increasingly expensive liability insurance, etc., have not been adequately compensated for by the DRG system – the new billing procedure under which a hospital is no longer paid according to patient days, but receives a specific flat rate per case for each illness.[3] Costs were also no longer adequately covered by more and more additional bureaucratic tasks in accounting, quality assurance and general documentation (a hospital doctor today spends almost 40% of his working time on bureaucracy and documentation). As a result, 15% of German hospitals are now in acute danger of insolvency and over 50% of German hospitals are in the red. This has led

---

3   The DRG system is a prospective, in fact a planned-economy financing model that no longer reimburses true costs based on need but instead sets an often unrealistic financing framework in advance of treatment that makes every elderly, critically ill patient with high care costs and a high risk of complications a threat to the bottom line.

to a growing takeover of municipal hospitals by hospital groups in recent years, so that 36% of municipal hospitals are now owned by groups. Due to the restrictive hospital financing in recent years, such a development was foreseeable, and one has to suspect that the creeping privatisation of the health system along American lines was secretly being pushed forward by politicians.

Now, of course, the municipal hospitals are not taken over by the corporations for charitable purposes, but these mostly listed companies pay out returns of 10-40% to their shareholders. These additional funds, which are taken away from the health system through profits, have further aggravated the situation and forced the hospitals more and more under the pressure of an economic competitive logic. The additional profits now generated naturally had to be recouped through corresponding savings; this usually involves terminating collective agreements, reducing staff and hiring cheap auxiliary staff, selecting treatment procedures according to profitability criteria, abolishing company pension schemes and outsourcing services to the low-wage sector. In North Rhine-Westphalia, for example, hospital staffing was reduced by 7.2% from 1995–2010, while the number of inpatients rose from 3.7 to 4.2 million, an increase of 13.5%. In addition, as a result of the demographic development, the so-called case mix index rose; this is an index that indicates the severity of an illness. Due to the ageing of the population, the amount of care required for old patients with several concomitant diseases is increasing. All these cost-cutting measures have led to an increase in the workload of the staff with a corresponding increase in the general stress level and a decline in job satisfaction.

The sickness rate among nursing staff in Germany is now 4.8%, while the national average is 3.36%; the absence of nurses due to illness is thus about 40% higher than the national average, whereby hospital staff very often also go to work sick, which is called presenteeism – 56% of hospital staff go to work despite illness. According to official figures, there is currently a shortage of 70,000 nursing staff in Germany. In Germany there are 9 nurses per 1000 inhabitants; in Norway there are 32. This is not because Norway has more money, but because of a different value weighting in health care expenditure.

In 2006, for example, the University Hospital Giessen Marburg was sold to Rhön AG. I quote from Wirtschaftswoche April 2016; under the headline 'Speculating with clinics – the financial disaster of German hospitals' it says here:

> Whoever sells their hospital to private owners, however, can expect angry citizens. Seven years after the state of Hesse sold the Gießen Marburg University Hospital to Rhön, the furore has not subsided. As a protest, the Elisabeth Church in Marburg, for example, regularly invites people to Monday prayers on health policy. In the Gothic church from the 13th century, it is said that it was often as full on these occasions as it otherwise was only at Christmas.

According to a *Spiegel* article from July 2013, doctors and nurses in Giessen Marburg complain of an extremely high workload. According to the management consulting institute McKinsey, the hospital is in danger of bankruptcy; meanwhile it needs an investment of 200 million Euros. Doctors' initiatives in Marburg are now also calling for the re-municipalisation of this university hospital. The problems are reminiscent of the so-called cross-border leasing deals, in which municipalities sold their water supply to foreign investors, for example, and were subsequently 'surprised' by huge financial problems.

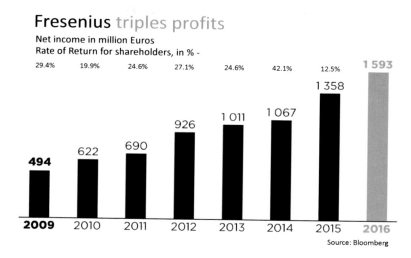

Figure 8 Fresenius profits

The chart in Figure 8 shows the development of profits at Fresenius, Europe's largest hospital group, which has now also acquired the aforementioned Rhön AG. Fresenius owns 112 hospitals in Germany alone. You can see the enormous growth in profits since 2009, here profits tripled by 2016 and now stand at 1.593 billion Euros. The top line shows the rate of return for investors; if you bought a Fresenius share in 2008 and sold it in 2009, you got a 29.4% return. In 2014, the return rose to 42.1%. We have to keep in mind that these funds come from contributions made by the insured to the statutory health insurance. Of the contributions paid by citizens for hospital care, between 20 and 30 % end up in the pockets of investors.

So basically, we are not dealing with a cost explosion, but with a reallocation of spending in the health care system. The savings, co-payments and personnel cuts in the health care system are in fact not savings measures as a result of a cost explosion, but rather the financing of increasing profits for the health care industry. This has been the real problem ever since politicians discovered healthcare as a market.

One could say that the economic logic in the health system is the problem it claims to solve. Instead of addressing the real, structural issues that lie in a parasitic, socially destabilising financial economy, the 'stroke rate' is increased following an industrial growth paradigm – 'an op has to run like a machine around the clock,' the managing director of the local clinic was recently quoted in the newspaper as saying, talking about the hospital's red figures.

'Boosting the economy' is a misplaced term in medicine. Hartmannbund, the professional association of German doctors, writes in its magazine 4/2016 p. 6, under the headline, *e-health is finally really taking off*. 'The digitalisation of the health market is picking up speed ever faster. According to a recent study, the management consultancy Roland Berger expects the global market volume to more than double from \$80 billion in 2015 to over \$200 billion by 2020.... More and more start-ups are entering the market with new business models, especially the segment with mobile services, such as smartphone apps, is driving the digitalisation of the industry with an annual growth of 40%.'

Programmes are shown on television where a computer program called IBM Watson (Apple and IBM have hired

2000 employees for the development of this program) as a 'digital colleague' surpasses the general practitioners in diagnostic accuracy and thus makes them look bad against the machine.[4] It is suggested with a cynicism that can hardly be surpassed that the art of healing is nothing more than data processing logic. Here, the increasing lack of relationship between doctor and patient in the economic gears is also sold as an increase in efficiency or as patient emancipation – Mammon has many faces! Instead of urgently needed, better care structures – in nursing, care for the elderly, midwifery, relief for single mothers, etc. – contributions to health care are being wasted on more and more pointless digital nonsense.

If you declare health care a market, don't be surprised if the money is missing where the profits have been skimmed.

One could also say: the financing of health care is increasingly moving away from people, away from direct support, nursing, advice, care – towards products, including financial products. The health care industry is now the largest industry in all industrialised countries worldwide. Before 1970, the care of the sick was largely a self-evident social good, just as kindergartens, schools, town halls, courts, etc. are. A hospital did not have to make a profit any more than a kindergarten or a public authority. With the beginning of the deregulation of the financial markets, the immense funds from health care now suddenly came into the sights of an economic strategy; 340 billion Euros per year in Germany

---

4   Editor's note: In the meantime IBM has sold its Watson Health assets to private equity firm Francisco Partners. Many other software players have now entered the healthcare software 'market', such as Google, Microsoft, Oracle and Amazon.

alone are a lucrative pot for investors. Thus, more and more money from health insurance contributions comes into the possession of profit-oriented companies, whereby ever higher profits are taken out of the health market. This is why everything that has to do with health and medicine costs many times more.

The pharmaceutical industry

This brings us to the now disastrous image of the pharmaceutical industry, whose business practices are increasingly taking on Mafia-like features. Literature critical of the pharmaceutical industry now fills entire libraries, but the public and, above all, politicians are still not quite aware of this, otherwise we would have had an uprising long ago. In 2015, the turnover of pharmaceutical companies worldwide amounted to 960 billion US dollars, with profits of around 250 billion dollars, which is almost twice the global expenditure on development aid (131 billion). This industry has the largest profit margins of any industry, averaging 20–30%! For example, the sales of the ten largest pharmaceutical companies in 2012 were $359 billion, with profits of $95 billion, a profit margin of 26.5%. Pfizer, one of the largest pharmaceutical giants in the U.S. generated sales of 51.6 billion in 2013, distributing 22 billion to shareholders, a profit of 43%. The actual task of the pharmaceutical industry, research, is increasingly being neglected; in the meantime, corporations spend on average only 10–15% of their sales on research and development. By contrast, spending on marketing is between 50 and 55%. In the USA, pharmaceutical companies spend an average of $5,000 per physician per year on advertising – it is not difficult to guess what such 'advertising' looks like.

Most of the active ingredients are imported by the pharmaceutical companies from the Far East, with the cost share of the active ingredients in the sales price averaging 1–2%. Again, we must have in mind that all these immense profits were originally contributions of citizens to health insurance, which are now disappearing into the pockets of shareholders and speculators from all over the world.

In an interview with Deutschlandradio Kultur, the author of the book *Bittere Pillen* ('Bitter Pills'), Hans Weiss, made the following statement (Weiss, 2007):

I got to know the second face of the pharmaceutical industry with my own eyes and ears. For example, for the book 'Corrupt Medicine' I posed as a pharma consultant, which is an industry consultant in the pharmaceutical field, I invented a company name – Solutions – and I registered for pharma-internal congresses. I paid for the invitation, three days of participation in a congress at just under €4,000, which is a lot of money, but everything is just expensive in the pharmaceutical industry. And when they pay that much money, nobody asks who they are, what they do, they are completely unsuspicious. There were about 500 top people from the pharmaceutical industry among themselves, no public, no journalists, about 30 top pharmaceutical managers from Germany, and then they hear quite blunt truths, such as: 'We throw up a marketing mix in the face of the doctors, and the amazing thing is, they swallow it!'

In order not to be subjected to the tiresome cliché of the conspiracy theorist, I would like to let a few renowned insiders have their say. Peter Gøtzsche is a Danish medical researcher and was director of the Nordic Cochrane Centre at the Ringshospital in Copenhagen until 2018. He had worked in the pharmaceutical industry for a long time. The Cochrane

Collaboration, as it was originally called, has been one of the largest pharma-independent medical research institutes. It collects medical research data and studies from all over the world, prepares meta-analyses for them and evaluates them according to certain evidence criteria. Peter Gøtzsche is therefore one of those who has an overview of the world-wide medical business like few others. Towards the end of his career, he summarised his experiences in a book with the provocative title *Deadly Medicine and Organized Crime – How Big Pharma Has Corrupted Healthcare* (Gøtzsche, 2013) Some might consider this title an exaggeration, but it quotes, for example, the former vice president of Pfizer, the world's largest pharmaceutical company:

> The resemblance of this industry to organized crime is frightening. The Mafia makes outrageous money, so does this industry. The side effects of organized crime are murders and deaths, and so are the side effects of this industry. The Mafia bribes politicians and other people, the pharmaceutical companies do the same.

There are many examples in the book where the pharmaceutical industry has tried to cover up dangerous and deadly side effects of their products at the cost of thousands of lives.

Convictions of Pharmaceutical Companies for Fraud, 2009-2012*

Company	Amount fined
Pfizer 2009	2.3 billion dollars
Novartis 2010	423 million dollars
Sanofi-Aventis 2009	95 million dollars
GlaxoSmithKlinen 2011	3 billion dollars
AstraZeneca 2010	520 million dollars
Johnson & Johnson 2012	1.1 billion dollars
Merck 2007	670 million dollars
Eli Lilly 2009	1.4 billion dollars
Abbot 2012	1.5 billion dollars

Source: Peter C. Götzsche, *Deadly Medicine and Organized Crime – How Big Pharma Has Corrupted Healthcare*, Routledge, 2013

* A small selection – the full list is much longer extending over many years

Figure 9 Convictions of pharmaceutical companies

Figure 9 shows a partial list of fines of up to $3 billion per year that individual corporations have had to pay between 2007–2012 for fraud, illegal marketing, counterfeiting, bribery, deception and profiteering. When one considers the calculations and profit margins of this industry, it becomes obvious that crimes are routinely booked here as business expenses in the sense of a calculated and organised crime. Another intimate connoisseur and highly renowned critic of the scene is Marcia Angell, who for 20 years was editor-in-chief of the *New England Journal of Medicine*, one of the world's most important medical journals. She teaches social medicine at Harvard University and in 2004 published her book entitled *The Truth About the Drug Companies: How They Deceive Us and What to Do About It.* (Angell, 2004). A quote from the book:

> It is simply no longer possible to believe much of the clinical research that is published, or to rely on the judgment of trusted physicians or authoritative medical guidelines. I take no pleasure in this conclusion, which I reached slowly and reluctantly over my two decades as an editor of the *New England Journal of Medicine*...

In her book, Angell demonstrates in great detail how pharmaceutical companies fleece patients, how they pocket the rewards of beneficial inventions made by others or sell as supposed innovation what in fact already exists. In particular, she cautions that oversight by politicians no longer works.

In 2009, the international pharmacology journal *Prescrire* subjected 109 newly approved drugs to analysis: it was found that of these 109 drugs, only three could be classified as minor therapeutic innovations, 76 of these drugs brought nothing new and 19 were considered health risks.

One of the suspicious marketing strategies of the pharmaceutical companies is the redefinition of healthy to sick people by lowering the threshold values for various measured values more and more. In the 1970s, the limit for a healthy blood glucose value was 144, the limit for cholesterol between 280 and 300, and for blood pressure 100 plus age was considered normal. In the meantime, all these limits have been successively lowered, creating millions of new patients. Today, a blood glucose level of over 100 is considered pre-diabetes. The cholesterol limit has been lowered to 200 mg/dl, which means that in Germany alone 70% of people over 40 have been declared patients. The medicines for lowering cholesterol levels, which are questionable in many respects, are now one of the top-selling drugs worldwide. The situation is similar with blood pressure, where we now have a limit of 120 over 80, turning 30–45% of the European population into risk patients in need of treatment.

Even completely normal phenomena in the human life course such as climacteric, crises with mood swings, baldness and potency disorders in old age, etc., have meanwhile been redefined as diseases with corresponding sales markets. In the committees that, for example, define guidelines and treatment standards for such 'new diseases,' it is not uncommon to find physicians with lucrative consulting contracts from those companies that profit from them.

These and many other measures have contributed to the increasing medicalisation of the population. Today, many things are treated pharmacologically that actually have psychosocial and structural social causes, such as the loneliness of old people. In a Swedish study[5], in which 762 nursing home residents were examined with regard to their use of medication, it was found that 67% take more than 10 different medications. In Germany, the ratios are similar; those over 80 take an average of 9.3 tablets per day. Among nursing home residents, 33% took three or more psychotropic drugs, 50% took antidepressants and tranquillizers, and 30% took so-called anticholinergics for incontinence. All these drugs can cause cognitive impairment, confu-

5   Kragh A. *Läkartidningen* 2004; 101: 994–9.

sion and falls as a result of dizziness and light-headedness, which in turn significantly increases mortality due to fractures. The consequences of these drug cocktails, which can no longer be calculated in terms of their effects and side effects, are then often misinterpreted as dementia. It is part of basic pharmacological knowledge that more than five different medications per day lead to interactions between the individual active ingredients that are unknown and can no longer be calculated. When more than five medications are taken per day we speak by definition of polypharmacy because we are taking an unjustifiable risk for the patient. In an article about the dangers of polypharmacy a typical case history was described, as I have experienced it all too often in over 30 years of clinical work.

> When my father was 88 he was hospitalised because he suffered from dizzy spells since he was taking more medication. In the hospital, he was given even more medication. As a result, he became confused and anxious and spoke incoherently. Then his doctor transferred him to a nursing home, where he soon appeared unkempt, crying and asking people to hold his hand. They categorised him as 'do not resuscitate' – and gave him more medication. I persuaded the doctor at the home to stop all medications and hired a self-employed nurse to feed my father organic food – rich in fruits, vegetables, grains, beans, nuts and seeds. After three days, my father experienced such a dramatic improvement that the nurses at the home didn't recognise him. When I called to talk to my father, he was himself again. He said he was bored and wanted to play cards. The next day he was discharged. He died several years later, peacefully relaxing at home. (Mann, 2009)

A major reason for polypharmacy is also the fear of doctors to discontinue a drug, because in times of increasing legal repression they arm themselves against possible accusations of 'omission'. Especially from younger colleagues, the sentence 'you'd better keep taking it, then we're on the safe side...' can often be heard. The tenor of court rulings in medical procedures often places therapeutic actionism above prudence; anyone who operates on 90 appendices out of a hundred for nothing because there was no appendicitis at all, or anyone who sends a patient into chronic intoxication with the 15th drug or even kills him, will not be legally prosecuted for having done something or for having treated in accordance with guidelines. Giovanni Maio speaks in this context of the prejudice of doing – the main thing is that one has acted, even if the measure is beyond all medical sense. In particular, the many nonsensical and severely stressful chemotherapies for advanced tumour diseases, which are usually sold as the 'last hope' or 'only chance' out of helplessness and speechlessness in the face of the inevitable, should also be mentioned here.

'We estimate that 58,000 patients per year die in internal medicine departments due to adverse drug reactions,' commented Prof. Dr. Jürgen Fröhlich, Director of the Department of Clinical Pharmacology at the Hannover Medical School, on what is now the third most common cause of death in Germany.

Another expert familiar with the subject is Dr Richard Horton, editor of *The Lancet*, another world-renowned medical journal:

> Much of the scientific literature, perhaps half, may simply be untrue. Afflicted by studies with small sample sizes, tiny effects, invalid exploratory analyses, and flagrant conflicts

of interest, together with an obsession for pursuing fashion-able trends of dubious importance, science has taken a turn towards darkness... No one is willing to take the first step toward restoring the integrity of the system.

80–90% of pharmacological studies are now funded or supported by the pharmaceutical industry, with only what promises profit being published accordingly. Christian Kreiß, an economics professor from Aalen, has described the massive threat to free research in his book *Gekaufte Forschung: Wissenschaft im Dienst der Konzerne* ('Bought research: Science in the service of corporations') (Kreiß, 2015). A worrying problem are the conflicts of interest in the entire industry. On the committees that develop treat-ment guidelines and therapy standards for numerous diseas-es, issuing them as general recommendations to the medical profession, there are people who are financially involved with the pharmaceutical companies.

Covert corruption

There is now an area that is referred to as 'covert corruption' in the healthcare sector. Let us take an example: The president of the Association of Senior Hospital Doctors (Leitenden Krankenhausärzte Deutschlands) in Germany, Dr. Hans-Fred Weiser, together with the Medical Association, examined the current employment contracts with chief physicians. A finding: one out of two contracts for new chief physicians today contains so-called bonus clauses. These are target agreements, as common in industry; if, for example, the number of operations for hip prostheses is increased by twenty percent, the annual salary of the chief physician increases accordingly. I know the case of a former colleague who accepted a senior position as a surgeon. He is known to me as a very careful diagnostician who, for example, very rarely performed an unnecessary appendectomy because his ultrasound diagnostic skills were highly reliable. This has now led to a significant reduction in the number of unnecessary appendectomies at his new employer, whereupon he received a reminder from the management, which is staffed with business economists – i.e. medical laymen – that he should ensure, in the economic interests of the hospital, that such forms of abdominal pain are operated on more generously.

The term 'consulting agreements' refers to agreements that pharmaceutical companies make with medical opinion leaders such as senior physicians and professors, who have a great influence on the recommendation of drugs. A chief physician, for example, often receives a high four-digit sum for a 45-minute lecture in which the efficacy of a certain drug is presented in a positive light.

These forms of covert corruption also include so-called 'user observations'. In these cases, physicians are encouraged by pharmaceutical representatives to prescribe specific medications, and they usually record their observations of the effects and side effects of these medications on an online form.[6] They then receive a fee per completed form or per patient, which averages €669 per doctor per patient. In 2014, a total of 16,952 physicians in Germany conducted such user observations, which corresponds to about 10% of physicians in private practice. Such practices are relatively common among oncologists in particular, as chemotherapies generate very high revenues; one infusion of chemotherapy costs around €1000. According to Professor Windeler of the Institute for Quality Assurance and Scientific Research in Health Care (IQWIG),[7] the data collected in this way are scientifically meaningless and cannot be used. In any case, every doctor is obliged to document side effects and report them to the manufacturer. 'Transparency International' has also long called for a ban on such practices.[8]

The term 'referral cartels' refers to agreements that doctors make with each other in order to selectively refer private

6   http://www.spiegel.de/gesundheit/diagnose/zahlungen-an-aer-zte-der-nette-pharmareferent-a-1104739.html:)
7   Institut für Qualitätssicherung und Wissenschaftlichkeit im Ge-sundheitswesen (IQWIG) in Germany
8   http://www.badische-zeitung.de/gesundheit-ernaehrung/warum-be-kommen-aerzte-geld-fuer-wertlose-pharma-studien

patients to each other, whereby very often unnecessary examinations are performed. Patients often have to travel enormous distances for this purpose or are sent to distant hospitals, which usually means an unnecessary additional burden and stress for patients and their relatives. This is usually sold to patients with the argument that they are being sent to a 'specialist'.

> The highest asset that medicine has as a profession is its trustworthiness. A doctor is still held in very high esteem, and it was precisely the monetary uninfluenceability of the medical profession that gave it prestige and privileges. It is irresponsible to call into question this monetary uninfluenceability through bonus payments! Therefore, a radical decoupling of the doctor's salary from his therapeutic decisions needs to be striven for, because only those doctors can show backbone who do not need to squint at their income.
>
> Giovanni Maio

The more doctors are urged to do something for a reward, the more meaningless they will find their profession in the long run. Self-interest and profit in particular always ultimately destroy the physician's self-respect. The more incentive systems are created, the more market-rational thinking grows. Such incentive systems undermine what should be the self-evident motivation: helping the other person.

The business with fear

People only think about drugs and vaccines; there is no profit in nutrition....

Luc Montaigner, Nobel Prize winner

Huge revenues can be generated with fear. Fear-mongering is an ideal instrument for enforcing economic and political interests – fear-mongering is *the* mass media suggestion technique par excellence. Every advertisement and every political propaganda calculates with the fears of humans – fear of illness, violence and death. But the most sophisticated technology makes use of the fear of exclusion, of being abandoned, the fear of not belonging anymore. '*If you don't have this smartphone you don't belong anymore and if you don't wear this brand you are out*'... are the hidden messages. Social devaluation and disintegration is the worst mortification for human beings, the fear of it is greater than of death. This is what advertising uses. In power management today, we talk about soft power,[9] which means that today you don't need to force people to do something by force. Most people are not yet armed against the subtleties of modern psychotechniques and suggestion strategies and can be manipulated more easily than they are usually aware. A lot of education still needs to be done in this area to free ourselves from this form of control.

---

9   See Prof. Rainer Mausfeld videos on YouTube. See also the websight for the Behaviour Insight Team, https://www.bi.team, their know-how used by corporations and governments internationally.

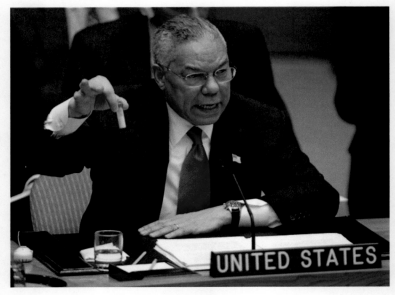

Figure 10

Figure 10 shows the former US Secretary of State Colin Powell in 2003 in front of the World Security Council, where he is handling a tube during a speech which supposedly contains a highly dangerous weapon of mass destruction from Iraq. As it later turned out, this was used to stir up a completely unfounded fear, which ultimately helped legitimise the American invasion of Iraq resulting in the deaths of hundreds of thousands of people. John Mearsheimer, a well-known U.S. political scientist at the University of Chicago, commented on this action by saying, *'Fear-mongering has played a major role in the last 70 years of American foreign policy.'*

Such propaganda techniques can also be impressively studied in the panic epidemics that are sparked almost every year, in which the fear of dangerous viruses is stirred up. 'Two million dead US citizens are to be feared!' With this threat, George W. Bush and his colleague Donald Rumsfeld put pressure on the American Senate to purchase the highly controversial flu drug Tamiflu for a total of 2 billion dollars as a 'precautionary' measure. The wave of fear also spilled over into Europe. Everywhere in the media people in protective suits could be seen disposing of masses of dead birds. Now the bird flu is a phenomenon which has been known for over 100 years and, as a flu epidemic, causes a certain mortality rate every year, just as it does in humans. Previously, these H5N1 viruses had been detected in isolated cases in people suffering from influenza, but the causal relationship between the virus and the severity or lethality of the flu courses could not be proven in any way. The panic was completely unjustified from a virological point of view. Nevertheless, within a few months Tamiflu generated a worldwide turnover of 6 billion dollars. The main beneficiary of the action was Donald Rumsfeld himself, who made many millions of dollars in profit as the main shareholder of the distributor company Gilead Science. Huge stockpiles of Tamiflu were created throughout Europe in the process (as in Figure 11).

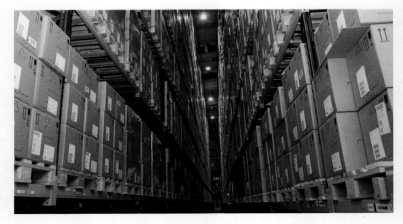

Figure 11 Tamiflu stockpiles in Great Britain

In the Süddeutsche Zeitung of 10th April 2014, under the headline *Sargnagel für Tamiflu* ('Nail in the coffin for Tamiflu'), one could read: 'Finally the long withheld data for Tamiflu are accessible. Their analysis shows: the influenza drug, which is stored in millions, is even less useful than thought and is even potentially harmful. Scientists attest to multi-organ failure by those responsible.' This was preceded by a years-long dispute between the *British Medical Journal* and the manufacturing company because the latter had refused to release the data that was supposed to prove the efficacy of the substance – a scandal of the first order! Millions of people are supposed to take a drug whose proof of efficacy or side-effect profile is kept secret! It was only when the English journal put the correspondence with the company on the internet in an 'Open Data Campaign' that the company sort of buckled and had to release the study data and documents that now confirmed the ineffectiveness of this drug. The facts were so clear and the amount of

46

money wasted so great that the Cochrane Network and the *British Medical Journal* decided to take an unusual step: they issued an urgent appeal to governments and health politicians worldwide at the same time as the 550-page review article was published containing all the evidence for Tamiflu's lack of efficacy.

The next wave of panic was swine flu in 2009, but by now people had become somewhat sensitised and sceptical as the urgent call for mass vaccination was heeded by very few. Vaccines worth a total of 130 million Euros had to be destroyed later as hazardous waste.

The sensationalist media usually encouraged these panic scenarios uncritically, because of course it was a way to make money. On 20 October 2009 the *Bild* newspaper ran the headline, 'Professor fears 35,000 deaths in Germany!' A few days earlier a young patient was shown in his hospital bed allegedly almost dying of swine flu. As it turned out, he had previously suffered a total collapse on the Ballermann beach in Majorca after presumably excessive partying or binge drinking, and the swine flu virus was detected in his blood. A few days later the Bild newspaper again reported that 'Infections explode!' At that time a total of two people had died, both of whom had serious pre-existing illnesses, whereby it was completely unclear whether the alleged swine flu virus was the cause or merely a side effect of the illness.

A scientifically brilliant and extremely detailed analysis of the business with epidemics has been presented by the Kiel internist Claus Köhnlein and the journalist Thorsten Engelbrecht in the book, Viruswahn ('Virus Mania'). With a considerable amount of hard factual material, the authors show that the hypotheses on the worldwide virus panic epidemics are factually not provable and partly also contradictory. At the same time they convincingly show that it is usually other causes such as drugs, medication, poor nutrition, stress, pesticides and heavy metals that severely damage or even completely destroy people's immune systems. Such circumstances are found exactly where the victims are. In this highly informative book, well-known and renowned virologists also comment on the importance of viruses, for example in AIDS. (Engelbrecht and Köhnlein, 2020[10])

Luc Montaigner, who received the Nobel Prize in 2008 for the discovery of the AIDS virus, also had this to say:

> Even after the greatest efforts and with the help of electron microscope images of cell cultures in which HIV is supposed to be present, it has not been possible to make particles visible that are typical of retroviruses in terms of their morphology....
>
> A healthy lifestyle and a healthy diet can cure an HIV infection completely without medication...
>
> If you build up the immune system of a poor African who is infected, I think he can then also get rid of HIV naturally. This is important knowledge that is completely ignored. People only think about drugs and vaccines; there is no profit in nutrition....

Many authors have repeatedly criticised the commercial links between the World Health Organisation (WHO) in

---

10 Editor's note: In the German edition of this book, Hardtmuth cites the original German 2010 edition of Engelbrecht and Köhnlein, which has since been updated and published in English, July 2020, to include Corona/COVID-19 in the sub-title. The updated English version is given in the References section.

Geneva and the pharmaceutical industry. The world's most important centre of health organisation and disease control entered into a so-called public–private partnership with industry years ago. 75% of the World Health Organisation's finances come from industry funding. The total budget of the WHO is about 4 billion dollars, 3 billion of which come from an industrial complex behind the Bill Gates Foundation with its 'Global Alliance for Vaccines and Immunisation', which in turn floods the African continent with vaccines and medicines. Instead of addressing the real structural problems, additional sales markets are being created here. The majority of African health problems are due to poverty, poor nutrition and lack of education – this is where the real help should start.

Salutogenesis

In the 1970s, the American sociologist Aaron Antonowski developed the so-called salutogenesis model, which initiated a change of perspective in medical thinking. The view expanded from the one-sided pathogenesis thinking – i.e. the question of what makes us ill – to the completely new question of what actually keeps us healthy. Previously, the pathogenesis theory mainly focused on external stressors such as viruses, bacteria, pollutants, toxins, allergens, etc. as causes of illness. In the meantime, we know that it is essentially inner health factors such as an intact immune system, resilience (emotional resilience), intact social bonds, good self-regulation and lifestyle, coping (ability to cope with problems), humanity, nutrition, hygiene and much more that are the mainstay of our health. The better these individual health factors are developed, the less danger there is from viruses and bacteria.

Epidemics are usually the result of poor living conditions: hunger, misery, war, fear, terror, poor nutrition and hygiene. In an intact and humane civil society, epidemics are practically non-existent. Functioning, vital societies with a living culture are far less susceptible to collective diseases and neuroses. The danger from viruses and bacteria is completely overrated by our profit-oriented health industry; viruses and bacteria are co-factors in the disease process, but not the sole cause.

Model of Salutogenesis

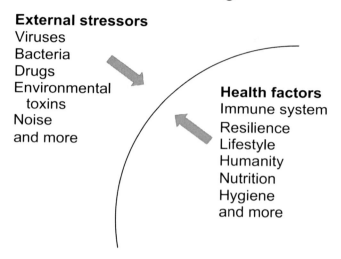

Figure 12 Salutogenesis Model

The role of viruses and bacteria in nature is still largely misunderstood; only 1% of these micro-organisms are even known or researched, they play a far greater role for our health and for the stability of ecological systems than they do for diseases – they only become significant as pathogens where salutogenic resources are correspondingly weakened. In the context of the health market, they represent an important propaganda tool for fear-mongering; a huge industry lives from the 'enemy image of microbes'. An excess of antibiotics, disinfectants in households, vaccinations and fever-reducing medicines, even for small children, has permanently irritated the immune systems in industrialised countries, so that we are now dealing with a flood of allergic and autoimmune diseases in the Western world.

With regard to the salutogenesis model, we would like to refer to an important study that was conducted between 1994 and 2014. In this so-called EPIK study (European Prospective Investigation into Cancer and Nutrition), more than 500,000 people were examined over a period of 20 years. First, their health status and lifestyle were determined and then they were observed over 20 years to see how corresponding diseases developed. The result was that a healthy lifestyle alone – physical activity, a healthy diet, normal body weight and not smoking – can reduce the risk of chronic disease by 78% overall: 93% less diabetes, 81% less heart attacks, 50% less strokes and 36% less cancer. If we could also reduce the negative stress and the many psychosocial stress factors in our hectic performance-oriented societies and ensure a balanced social climate and successful social interaction, we would all be much healthier.

Social justice and health

There is a connection between social justice and health that has been documented in numerous studies. Although this connection is not yet fully understood, the data is convincing. The more privilege and profit thinking prevail in a society, the greater the income disparities, the more unjust this society becomes and the more unhealthy people are. Unjust societies with a strong social divide promote existential fears, competition, envy, resentment, exclusion and experiences of not being valued; the psychosocial experience of degradation and disintegration is a widely underestimated disease factor. In social medicine we speak of gratification crises when, for example, people make an effort at work, are committed and perform far beyond the required level without receiving the corresponding social recognition and the feeling of livelihood security in return.

Figure 13 below shows the development of income inequality in the USA and Europe from 1900–2010. Again, we encounter our red arrow here, which marks the beginning of the deregulation of financial markets. From this point on inequality rises steeply, especially in the USA.

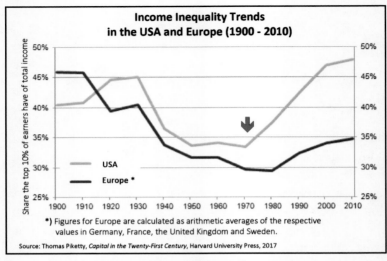

Figure 13 Income inequality trends

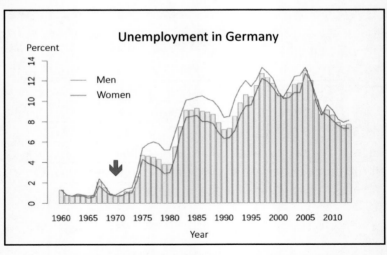

Figure 14 Unemployment in Germany

What are the social ramifications for the increasing income inequality trends?

In Figure 14 we see the development of unemployment in Germany since 1960; here, too, a steep rise or the beginning of mass unemployment can be seen at the beginning of the 1970s (red arrow).

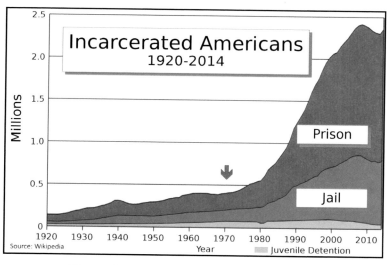

Figure 15 Incarceration trends in the USA

In Figure 15 we see a huge increase in incarcerated Americans from the same period, with the red band showing total penitentiary inmates in federal prisons, the blue those in state jails and the light blue representing the number of incarcerated juvenile Americans.

If we compare incarceration figures for different countries, it appears to have a close relationship to the levels of income inequality. This is illustrated in Figure 16, with inequalities based on income gaps as shown in Figure 17.

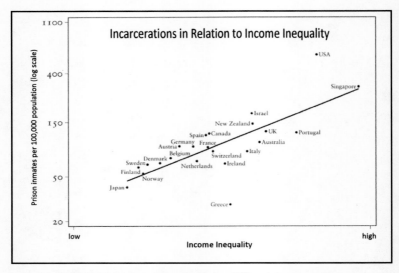

Figure 16 Incarcerations in different countries

Figure 17 shows the income differences between the top and bottom 20% of the population in Europe, as well as in the USA and Singapore. In Japan the difference in income between the richest and poorest 20% is about four times, while in the USA this gap shows a further doubling. The countries with the smallest gap between rich and poor are Japan and the Scandinavian countries. What is remarkable is that these countries have largely non-privatised health care systems, which instead of being performance-based – those who pay a lot get a lot – are oriented towards needs-based health care, i.e. everyone gets what they need.

Against this background, we now look at the connection between income inequality and certain health parameters.

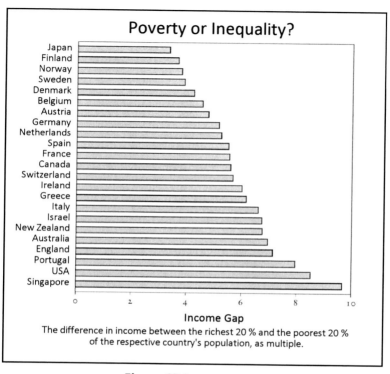

Figure 17 Income gaps

The relationship between inequality of distribution and life expectancy is shown in Figure 18. On this and the following graphs income inequality is shown on the horizontal X-axis and the corresponding health parameters on the vertical one. Japan and the Scandinavian countries perform best in terms of life expectancy. Of the European countries, Portugal and the United Kingdom have the greatest income inequality, and life expectancies here are in the lower range. The average life expectancy of Americans, at 78.94 years, is significantly lower than in Japan, for example (83.59 years).

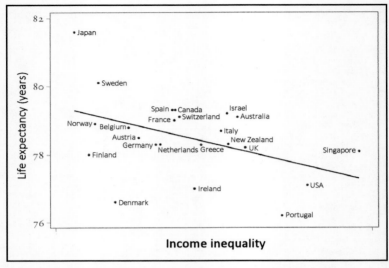

Figure 18 Life expectancy and income inequality

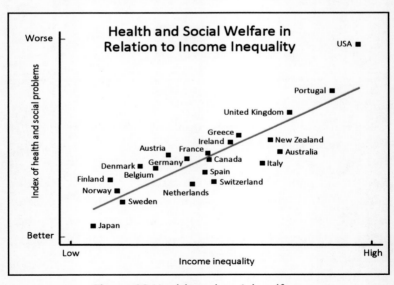

Figure 19 Health and social welfare

Figure 19 shows the relationship between general health and social problems and income inequality. Again, the problems occur significantly more often in countries where the income gap is wide open.

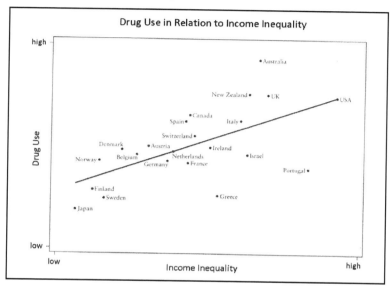

Figure 20 Drug use in relation to income inequality

Figure 20 shows a relationship between drug use and income inequality; here Australia performs particularly poorly, as do the USA, United Kingdom and New Zealand.

The USA is also far ahead of all other countries in terms of homicides per 1 million inhabitants; here, there are more than 60 homicides per year per 1 million inhabitants, compared to about one-sixth in Germany and the Scandinavian countries. Its relationship to income inequality is considered in Figure 21.

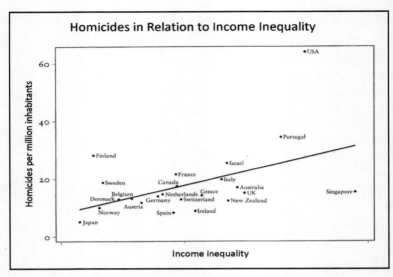

Figure 21 Homicides in relation to income inequality

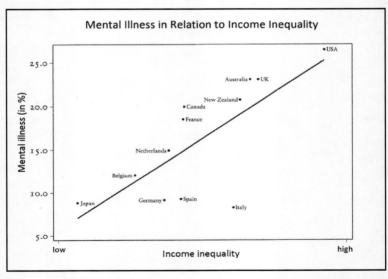

Figure 22 Mental illness in relation to income inequality

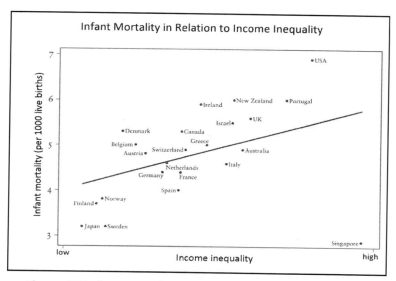

Figure 23 Infant mortality in relation to income inequality

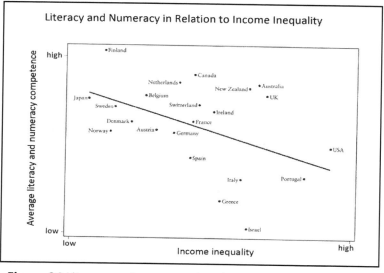

Figure 24 Literacy and numeracy in relation to income inequality

Mental illness also shows a similar distribution among the different countries in relation to income inequality (Figure 22). The same applies to infant mortality. (Figure 23)

In terms of school performance, countries with unbalanced social distribution are also lagging behind. The graph shows average performance in mathematics and literacy (Figure 24).

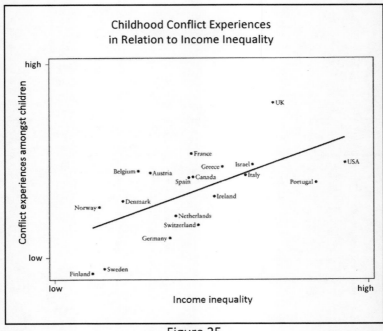

Figure 25

Figure 25 shows the relationship between children's experiences of conflict with income inequality. The statistics are based on the percentages of beatings, intimidation and bad experiences among peers.

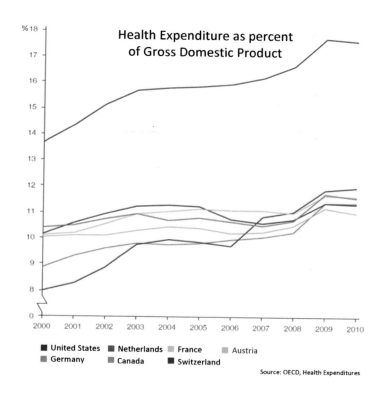

Figure 26 Health expenditure as percent of Gross Domestic Product

If we now look at the development of healthcare spending in the various countries, we see that the USA, with its largely privatised healthcare system, has by far the most expensive healthcare system in the world. The American population now spends more than 18% of its gross domestic product on health, which is in clear contrast to the poor overall health balance in this country. The light blue curve at the bottom of the graph shows the development of healthcare spending in Canada; here, similar to the Scandinavian countries, the healthcare system is mainly financed from tax revenues.

There is also a clear correlation with distributive justice in a society for illiteracy, obesity, trust among people and depression. These correlations were essentially worked out by health scientists and epidemiologists Kate Pickett and Richard Wilkinson from London (figures 16–25; see Wilkinson & Pickett, 2010). It must be emphasised that it is not average income but distributive justice that is relevant for the different levels of health in different countries. Basically, we do not need statistics to perceive that unjust societies foster more social tensions and existential anxieties, they generate more competitive pressures, exclusion, and more experiences of social decline and devaluation. Political radicalisation also stems essentially from a sense of social inferiority among the disadvantaged classes. In such societies, the individual is under constant social evaluation pressure at the expense of community and friendship ties. Wilkinson concludes that inequality makes a society socially dysfunctional.

Epilogue

'With the excessive economisation of medicine, the willingness of all actors to do something for the other without question and without pursuing an economic calculation is dwindling. This is precisely the re-evaluation of values by economics. The social question is replaced by the strategic question of profitability, which means nothing other than a mental monetisation of medical assistance.

The remuneration system financially punishes physicians who try to implement relationship medicine in the interest of their patients, and it rewards those who rely on technology and invasiveness instead of conversation.... As a result of the interplay between numbers-oriented medicine and calculating economics, everything for which numbers cannot be provided is currently deemed unnecessary.'

Giovanni Maio

The non-measurable things that actually make up a person are disappearing more and more from the sights of a calculating health economy.

Since the deregulation of the financial markets at the beginning of the 1970s, health care has also been distorted by the dictates of an all-dominant market logic to such an extent that it is increasingly in danger of losing sight of its actual core tasks. Since the 1970s, money as a legalised drug has unleashed an excessive, global capital frenzy, which mean-

65

while poses a serious threat not only to social world peace: all areas of life, nature and culture are increasingly permeated by the morbid stink of greed and avarice.[11] The social organism is becoming weaker and weaker, but the diagnosis of a global plague has not yet been made although the disease is progressing rapidly.

The cure can only lie in recalling the threefold nature of the social organism: freedom in intellectual life (liberté), equality in legal life (égalité) and fraternity in economic life (fraternité). Today, economic life overshadows the other spheres in a pathological way. Global financial capitalism clearly shows us the pathology of the social carcinoma, how it increasingly undermines our cultural organism and increasingly fuels warlike conflicts worldwide, as Henrik Paulitz cogently demonstrates in his book *Anleitung gegen den Krieg – Analysen und friedenspolitische Übungen* ('Manual against war – analyses and peace policy exercises', Paulitz, 2016).

What we need is complete transparency and open access to all relevant medical research data, because it affects us all. We need a radical decoupling of medical research from economic interests. The very fact that the organs of the health system – offices, ministries, research institutes, professional medical associations, etc. – are the institutions most frequently visited by lobbyists shows the overloading of medicine with external vested interests. Free research also requires free and independent journalism, which does not aim at quotas and circulation by serving sensationalism and

---

11 The drug 'money' fulfils all the criteria of an addictive disease: growing dependence and increasing need despite rising consumption, increase in tolerance, loss of other interests, loss of control, decline in moral values and acquisitive criminality, withdrawal symptoms.

mainstream clichés, but understands its profession in terms of responsibility for the truth and as a contribution to the development of a mature and enlightened civil society. The task of politics is to ensure that cultural and intellectual life remains independent and is not undermined or deformed by economic calculations.

For those who carry the Christian C on their flags, one may remind again and again that Jesus, the archetype of man, did not tolerate dealers and money-changers in the temple; it is the only place in the Bible where the Son of God becomes really angry and even uses a rod to chase the money-changers away.

The ethics of medical and nursing care and the Christian doctrine of salvation were, the further we look back in history, coming out of the same spirit, and so to this day the logic of profit has no place in a hospital or a consulting room.

Afterword

The logic of profit has no place in a hospital
or a consulting room.

Thomas Hardtmuth

Any cursory look at the field of modern medicine shows that, to misquote The Bard, 'something is decidedly rotten in the State of bio-pharmaceutical medicine'; and in this short book, Thomas Hardtmuth shines a searching light on some of the reasons why this might be so.

The term 'paradigm' is so overused these days that it's in danger of losing the gravity and power of its original meaning. Yet for those acquainted with Kuhnian paradigm theory (e.g. Kuhn, 1962; Cohen, 2015; Kidd & House, 2021), it appears that mainstream medicine is now so awash with contradictions, lacunae and corruption that humanity may well be on the verge of a fundamental and much-needed paradigm shift in our philosophies and practices around health, disease and well-being. What follows here should very much be seen in this light.

I wish to begin this Afterword to the welcome translation of Thomas Hardtmuth's German-language book by declaring an interest. Last year I co-wrote a book with Thomas titled *Beyond Mainstream Medicine* – so I am very familiar with his work and writings, and am perhaps some distance from being a disinterested observer! Notwithstanding my bias, I hope the following commentary will add to and embellish

68

what you have just read.

This short book is based on a lecture; and as such it is necessarily and unavoidably limited in the ground it can cover, and the complexity of the case it can make. In this invited afterword, therefore, I will seek to develop some of the implications for modern healthcare systems that stem from the strong critique of 'capitalistic medicine' offered in this book.

Capitalism and/in health care and the medical system

I will briefly mention a few key studies that, with Hardt-muth, strongly challenge capitalism in health care. Focusing on the USA, in *Health Care Under the Knife* Howard Waitzkin and the Working Group on Health Beyond Capitalism have given a comprehensive overview of the ills arising from the financialisation/capitalisation of health care, focusing on such issues as the 'proletarianisation' of health care employees, doctors' loss of control over health care, the high rates of burn-out, depression and suicide amongst physicians and health-care staff, the so-called 'medical industrial complex' and monopolisation tendencies in health care, and so on.

Donohoe (2020, p. 49) refers to 'the capitalist manifesto preached by "health care MBA" degree programs and weekend "health care business seminars"' – a sure indication of how medical trainings are saturated with a usually uncritical capitalist ideology that is rarely if ever questioned. There exists a substantial literature critiquing capitalism in health care (e.g. Navarro, 1976; Navarro & Berman, 1983; Boggs, 2005; Brezis, 2011; Lexchin, 2018; Benach et al.,

2019; Legge, 2019;), and a study drawing together all this literature is surely long overdue.

Science, 'scientific' medicine and their manifold vicissitudes

We should by no means assume that science itself is an unproblematic process that invariably reaches 'objective', disinterested conclusions (Feyerabend, 1978; Michaels, 2008; Lewis, 2014; Bausell, 2021) – nor, indeed, that '*the* science' is 'settled' (Condon, 2019). The latter viewpoint is fundamentally *un*scientific – and ignores the multitude of examples throughout history where the scientists of the day were convinced of the rightness of their ontology – only to have their certainty dismantled in the light of later scientific discoveries. In the realm of medicine itself, the corruption of science has also been extensively documented (e.g. Krimsky, 2003, 2019; McGarity & Wagner, 2008; Walker, 2001).

There are a number of other grave concerns about mainstream scientific medicine that I don't have the space to cover in any depth here: for example, general critiques of medicine and medical practices (e.g. Carlson, 1975; Illich, 1976; Taylor, 1979; Conrad & Schneider, 1992; Payer, 1992; Walker, 1993; Welch et al., 2011; Daniels, 2013; McCartney, 2013; Steganga, 2018; O'Mahony, 2019); the corruption of the pharmaceutical industry (Sidhwa, 1976; Lexchin, 1984; Collier, 1989; Payer, 1992; Abramson, 2004, 2022; Angell, 2004; Moynihan & Cassels, 2005; Dumit, 2012, Frances, 2013; Gøtzsche, 2013; Kenber, 2021); the phenomenon of iatrogenic (harm-causing) medicine (D'Arcy & Griffin, 1979; Sharpe & Faden, 1998; Last, 2008; Bigelsen, 2011;

Null, 2011; Dean, 2014; Lester & Parker, 2023); the field of (bio)medical research and evidence-based medicine (Krimsky, 2003, 2019; Kendrick, 2014; Patashnik et al., 2017; Steganga, 2018); medical ethics in modern biomedicine (Smith, 2016); the so-called 'medicalisation of society' (Misselbrook, 2001; Frances, 2013); the problematic relationship between technology and medical treatments (Reiser, 1978; Taylor, 1979; Gadamer, 1996; Cassels, 2012; Kaufman, 2105); the malign influence of corporations on public health (Freudenberg, 2014; Walker, 1993, 2017); the Audit Culture in health care (King & Moutsou, 2010; House, 2012); disreputable attacks on alternative medical treatments (Carter, 1992); the radically downplayed effectiveness of natural treatments and the healing power of illness (Sobel, 1979; Bland, 2014; Dethlefsen & Dahlke, 2016; Howick, 2017) – not to mention the huge and ever-growing literature on vaccine damage.

It would be lazy to claim that this litany of problematic issues – and the list could easily be extended – stem directly from the existence of capitalism in health care; yet it would also be difficult to argue that capitalism, broadly defined, is not at least *implicated* in some way in most of them. Criticism is easy, of course, and in what follows I will highlight some of the pioneering new initiatives that the current malaise in mainstream medicine is spawning, and which I think Hardtmuth would approve of.

Initiatives beyond bio-pharmaceutical capitalism

There are moves afoot globally, then, that are responding to the limitations and iatrogenic nature of bio-pharmaceutical medicine (cf. Jarman, 2022–3), and which are in the tradition of the salutogenic approach discussed by Hardtmuth. Here I will mention just five brief examples.

First, the UK **People's Health Alliance** (https://the-pha.org/) was founded in 2022, aiming to reduce the influence of Big Pharma, with the power of choice returned to the individual and championing a paradigm shift from treating disease to creating health. An organic, people-led approach to healthcare is the aim – as they proclaim on their website:

> We're here to facilitate your ideas, inspirations and creations within your local communities. We're about collaborations, connections and support…. We understand that health is far more than treating the symptoms of disease. We know that true health comes from taking an integrated approach, considering mind, body and spirit.

Advocating taking responsibility for personal health choices, the PHA encourages people to start viewing these choices as an investment in future health, inspiring people to shift their perceptions and mindset around healthcare. 'We have been conditioned to look outside of ourselves for too long…. It's time to reconnect with nature and all of the healing qualities it holds.' (website)

The PHA's ten principles include: 'Empower people to take responsibility for their own health'; 'Commit to self-improvement and learning new things'; and 'Embrace an integrated approach'. (website)

Secondly, in The Netherlands, there's **Buurtzog** – Revolutionising Home Care (www.buurtzorg.com). Buurtzorg Nederland was founded in 2006 by Jos de Blok and a team of professional nurses who saw years of 'reform' having undermined their relationships with patients. De Blok and colleagues set up Buurtzorg to look after people at home, in a way their values and craft demanded.

Each team of 10–12 nurses operates at the neighbourhood level (covering approximately 10,000 people and 40 patients), empowering nurses to go beyond the mere medical management of their patients. Buurtzorg's nurses are akin to 'health coaches' creating sustainable solutions leading towards prevention and care independence. Working closely with GPs, they organise all the supporting care, drawing in families, friends, and volunteers, seeing themselves as community-builders.

Thirdly, in Switzerland, **Anthrosana** (www.anthrosana.ch) is a patient-support organisation building on anthroposophical principles. It provides information on all aspects of health, illness and lifestyle, encouraging the use of complementary and especially anthroposophic medical treatments in Switzerland (e.g. Evans & Rodger, 1992; Steiner, 2013). Anthrosana is for everyone interested in a holistic approach that includes both mainstream and complementary medicine.

As fourth example, in the USA under the clinical leadership of Dr Peter McCullough, **The Wellness Company** (https://www.twc.health/) is based in Boca Raton, Florida. Founder and chairman Foster Coulson was responding to a demonstrably failing medical system, oppressive government health policies, and the lack of appreciation for natural approaches to cure illnesses. By unequivocally championing medical freedom and the right to affordable health care, the Wellness Company's vision strongly advocates for the right to make one's own medical choices. The company offers patient-centred medicine promising improved health outcomes, convenient access to physicians, and lower costs of healthcare for patients that is committed to affordability.

Lastly, **The World Council for Health (WCH)** (https://worldcouncilforhealth.org/) is a global coalition of health-focused initiatives and civil society groups which 'seeks to broaden public health knowledge and sense-making through science and shared wisdom.' Coalition partners 'are dedicated to safeguarding human rights and free will while empowering people to take control of their health and well-being.' (website)

Founded in May 2022 at the inaugural Better Way Conference in Bath, UK, there are now over 190 partner organisations from over 45 countries within the WCH coalition. As a reference point for partners, communities and individuals, the conference adopted their *7 Principles of a Better Way*: 1) We act in honour and do not harm; 2) We are free beings with free will; 3) We are part of nature; 4) Spirituality is integral to our well-being; 5) We thrive together; 6) We value different perspectives; and 7) We use technology with discernment. Through the coalition partners, the WCH provides extensive resources and hosts regular seminars on health and related issues. They state as a further principle (from their website):

> With courage, we do not tolerate:
> · The violation of people's inalienable rights and freedoms;
> · Profit, power and influence coming before the well-being of people and planet.

This is just a small selection of the post-pharmaceutical initiatives currently springing up across the globe, which promise to increasingly displace bio-pharmaceutical capitalism that has dominated the medical world for decades. The bottom-up re-education of ever more citizens about a holistic, non-mechanistic understanding of health and well-being will be key in this process, with an increasing proportion of people rejecting the symptom-centric pharmaceutical world-view and replacing it with a far more naturalistic, holistic one.

Health care and Rudolf Steiner's threefolding approach

It would be wrong to assume uncritically that because capitalism is not an appropriate means for delivering a sensible medical system, the only alternative is a state-socialist approach. An alternative approach that seeks a third way beyond both capitalism and socialism, and to which Hardtmuth refers at the end of his lecture, is Austrian spiritual polymath Rudolf Steiner's so-called 'threefolding approach' (see Masters, 2022a, b; the following explication relies heavily on Masters). A century ago, Steiner campaigned for a threefold approach that addressed the failures of both traditional capitalism and centralised state socialism. Masters maintains that the serious instances of fraud and lack of transparency that have recently come to light in the medical world could not have happened in the health system constructed on threefolding principles.

Steiner detailed the existence of three basic spheres of society – culture, politics and economics – maintaining that if each sphere could be guided by the celebrated ideals of *liberté, égalité, fraternité*, respectively, then societal functioning would be substantially enhanced. For Steiner, the *cultural realm* would ideally be guided by *liberté* – personal freedom – at all times. The *political realm* (concerned with rights and responsibilities alone) would be guided by *égalité*; and the *economic domain* works best when run in an *associative* manner (hence 'Associative Economics' – see Houghton Budd, 2003). Crucially, Steiner argued that the three realms – culture, politics and economics – should be kept largely independent (or relatively autonomous) from one another, with the three realms afforded a level of independence such that they are free from undue and inappropriate 'contamination' by each other.

Under a threefold approach to health care, scientific research (a part of the cultural domain in Steiner's definition) would be independent from both the State and industry (the economic domain). The pharmaceutical industry would not then be able unduly to influence the work of scientists or university departments; and governments would not be able to censor research findings to suit their partisan interests and narratives. As a result, then, inappropriate contamination between the three spheres of society would be radically reduced, and scientific and medical researchers would simply be interested in advancing knowledge, not looking over their shoulder in order to please funders or a State bureaucracy (Masters, ibid.).

Masters provides some highly prescient examples of the damage done to health care because of inappropriate 'contamination' between spheres. For example, in the Covid era, 'Vast numbers of doctors... have not baulked at giving healthy children novel gene "therapy" Covid jabs, despite them not being at risk from Covid, and despite there being

76

poor short-term safety data and no long-term safety data for these jabs' (Masters, 2022b).

A threefolding approach to health care would also curtail the situation whereby some of our most eminent physicians and academics are 'cancelled', bullied and threatened with the loss of professional licences and/or employment. Highly accomplished experts such as Dr Peter McCullough were raising major concerns about 'the Covid "science"', and yet others were able to threaten them via their connections to industry or politics. It would be difficult to find a more pernicious example of the contamination of one societal realm (culture) by the other two (economics and politics) (Masters, ibid.).

Masters also cites the US Food and Drug Administration's disturbing attempt to withhold, for 75 years, the number of deaths following Pfizer's jab trials – an example of the *political* realm being contaminated by the economic. The FDA represents the political realm in that it is supposed to protect the public, and the people's *right* not to be harmed. Yet with some 75 per cent of the FDA's drug review budget coming from Big Pharma, it's clear that inter-realm corruption between Steiner's three spheres is rife. Many more examples could be given, of course.

Under a 'common-sense' threefold approach, then, conflicts of interest such as these would be minimised, and proper foundations for truth, transparency and trust in public life would be far more effectively established. In the case of the UK National Health Service, according to Masters (2023), it does have some three-folding aspects – but not the heavy involvement of the State, nor its increasing commercialisation, which is moving in the opposite direction to authentic three-folding.

According to Masters (2023), in the free cultural sphere, the right to choose one medicine over another is central. He continues, 'Not only does the State not interfere with my consumption choices (whether of shoes or medicine), neither does the economic process judge what I see as my need. It just responds to it with the relevant production' (Masters, personal communication). Masters concludes, 'Might Steiner's model provide the magic key that critics of both traditional capitalism and centralised state socialism have long been seeking?'.

In conclusion

It was philosopher of science Paul Feyerabend who wrote tellingly about the authoritarian tendencies in modern science (Feyerabend, 1978; Kidd & House, 2021); and what has recently unfolded in the era of Covid certainly gives strong support to Feyerabend's grave concerns (e.g. Boyle, 2022; Ryder, 2021).

Thomas Hardtmuth's short book helpfully opens up a critical space in which all the issues covered in this Afterword (and more) can be discussed and interrogated. It would be unduly simplistic to place all of the ills of modern medicine at the door of 'capitalism'; yet capitalism and all that goes with it is surely *implicated* in some way in virtually all of the vicissitudes of the medical-pharmaceutical complex. The full story in all its intricacies is a highly complex one, and requires a study far more extended than is found here. Yet the perspective offered here by Hardtmuth will be an essential feature of any such elucidation.

We urgently have to find a better way with health, illness and well-being; and Thomas Hardtmuth is one of the voices we must listen to in order to fashion and then implement it.

Richard House

Stroud, March 2023

References

Abramson, J. (2004). *Overdosed America: The Broken Promise of American Medicine*. New York: HarperCollins.

Abramson, J. (2022). *Sickening: How Big Pharma Broke American Health Care and How We Can Repair It*. Boston, Mass.: Mariner Books.

Angell, M. (2004). *The Truth about the Drug Companies: How They Deceive Us and what to Do about It*. New York: Random House.

Bausell, R.B. (2021). *Problem with Science: The Reproducibility Crisis and What to Do about It*. Oxford: Oxford University Press.

Benach, J., Pericàs, J.M., Martínez-Herrera, E. & Bolíbar, M. (2019). Public health and inequities under capitalism: systemic effects and human rights. In J. Vallverdú, A. Puyol & A. Estany (eds), *Philosophical and Methodological Debates in Public Health* (pp. 163–80). Cham, Switzerland: Springer.

Bigelsen, H. (2011). *Doctors Are More Harmful than Germs: The Truth about Chronic Illness: How Surgery Can Be Hazardous to Your Health – and What to Do about It*. Berkeley, Calif.: North Atlantic Books.

Bland, J.S. (2014). *The Disease Delusion: Conquering the Causes of Chronic Illness for a Healthier, Longer, and Happier Life*. New York: Harper Wave.

Boggs, C. (2005). Review essay: Big Pharma and the corporate colonization of American medicine, *New Political Science*, 27 (3), pp. 407–21.

Boyle, F.A. (2022). *Resisting Medical Tyranny: Why the Covid-19 Mandates Are Criminal*. Cardiff-by-the-Sea, Calif.: Waterside Productions.

Braun, B., Kühn H. & Reiners, H. (1998). *Das Märchen von der Kostenexplosion – Populäre Irrtümer zur Gesundheitspolitik*

[The fairy tale of the cost explosion – Popular misconceptions about health policy]. Frankfurt: Fischer Verlag.

Brezis, M. (2011). Vulnerability of health to market forces, *Medical Care*, 49 (3), pp. 232–9.

Buchbinder, R. & Harris, I. (2021). *Hippocrasy: How Doctors Are Betraying Their Oath*. Sydney: NewSouth.

Carlson, R.J. (1975). *The End of Medicine*. New York: John Wiley.

Carter, J.P. (1992). *Racketeering in Medicine: The Suppression of Alternatives*. Charlottesville, VA: Hampton Road Publishing Co.

Cassels, A. (2012). *Seeking Sickness: Medical Screening and the Misguided Hunt for Disease*. Vancouver: Greystone Books.

Cohen, M. (2015). *Paradigm Shift: How Expert Opinions Keep Changing on Life, the Universe, and Everything*. Exeter: Imprint Academic.

Collier, J. (1989). *The Health Conspiracy: How Doctors, the Drug Industry and the Government Undermine Our Health*. London: Century Hutchinson.

Condon, B. (2019). *Science for Heretics: Why So Much of Science is Wrong*. ISBN 978-1-9164572-8.

Conrad, P. & Schneider, J.W. (1992). Medicine as an institution of social control. In their *Deviance and Medicalization: From Badness to Sickness* (pp. 240–60). Philadelphia: Temple University Press.

D'Arcy, P.F. & Griffin, J.P. (1979). *Iatrogenic Diseases*. Oxford: Oxford University Press.

Daniels, J. (2013). *The Lethal Dose: Why Your Doctor Is Prescribing It*. CreateSpace Independent Publishing Platform.

Dean, C. (2014). *Death by Modern Medicine: Seeking Safe Solutions,* 3rd edn. Perth, WA: Perfect Pitch Editions.

Dethlefsen, T. & Dahlke, R. (2016). *The Healing Power of Illness: Understanding What Your Symptoms Are Telling You*, 2nd edn. Boulder, Col.: Sentient Publications (orig. 1983).

Donohoe, M. (2020). Health care under the knife: moving beyond capitalism for our health (review of Waitzkin et al., 2018). *Social Medicine*, 13 (2), 48–54.

Dumit, J. (2012). *Drugs for Life: How Pharmaceutical Companies Define Our Health*. Durham, NC: Duke University Press.

Engelbrecht, T. & Köhnlein, C. (2020). *Virus Mania: Corona/ COVID-19, Measles, Swine Flu, Cervical Cancer, Avian Flu, SARS, BSE, Hepatitis C, AIDS, Polio. How the Medical Industry Continually Invents Epidemics, Making Billion-Dollar Profits at Our Expense*. Books-on-Demand. Also available in English as an Audible Audiobook.

Evans, M. & Rodger, I. (1992). *Anthroposophical Medicine: Healing for Body, Soul and Spirit*. London: Thorsons / HarperCollins.

Feyerabend, P. (1978). *Science in a Free Society*. London: Verso.

Frances, A. (2013). *Saving Normal: An Insider's Revolt against Out-Of-Control Psychiatric Diagnosis, DSM-5, Big Pharma, and the Medicalization of Ordinary Life*. New York: William Morrow.

Freudenberg, N. (2014). *Lethal but Legal: Corporations, Consumption, and Protecting Public Health*. New York: Oxford University Press.

Friedrich, M. & Weik, M. (2014). *Der größte Raubzug der Geschichte: Warum die Fleißigen immer ärmer und die Reichen immer reicher werden* [The greatest robbery in history: Why the hard-working are getting poorer and the rich are getting richer]. Bastei Lübbe, 7th edition.

Gadamer, H.-G. (1996). *The Enigma of Health*. Stanford, Calif.: Stanford University Press.

Gøtzsche, P. (2013). *Deadly Medicines and Organised Crime: How Big Pharma Has Corrupted Healthcare*. Boca Raton, Fla.: CRC Press.

Hardtmuth, T. (2015). Tiermast, Mikroorganismen und die Biologie der Moral. Kulturzeitschrift, in *Die Drei* (März).

Hardtmuth, T. & House, R. (2022). *Beyond Mainstream Medicine: Dialogue towards a New Paradigm for Health,* Stroud: InterActions.

Houghton Budd, C. (2003). *The Metamorphosis of Capitalism: Realising Associative Economics*. Canterbury / Turvey, Beds.: New Economy Publications.

House, R. (2012). General practice counselling amidst the 'audit culture': history, dynamics and subversion of/in the hypermodern National Health Service, *Psychodynamic Counselling*, 18 (1), pp. 51–70.

Howick, J. (2017). *Doctor You: Introducing the Hard Science of Self-Healing*. London: Coronet.

Illich, I. (1976). *Limits to Medicine: Medical Nemesis – The Expropriation of Health.* London: Marion Boyars.

Jarman, B. (2022–3). Where now with health? *New View* magazine, 106 (Jan–March), pp. 34–5.

Kaufman, S.R. (2105). *Ordinary Medicine: Extraordinary Treatments, Longer Lives, and Where to Draw the Line*. Durham, NC: Duke University Press.

Kenber, B. (2021). *Sick Money: Sky-high Prices and Dirty Tricks: Inside the Global Pharmaceutical Industry*. Edinburgh: Canongate.

Kendrick, M. (2014). *Doctoring Data: How to Sort out Medical Advice from Medical Nonsense*. Caldicor, Monmouthshire: Columbus Publishing.

Kidd, I.J. & House, R. (2021). 'We're all Feyerabendians now!': Where science and society meet – the contemporary relevance of Paul K. Feyerabend, 1924–94. *AHPB Magazine for Self & Society*, 6; available at https://tinyurl.com/ykpse3js).

King, L. & Moutsou, C. (eds). (2010). *Rethinking Audit Cultures: A Critical Look at Evidence-based Practice in Psychotherapy and Beyond*. Ross-on-Wye: PCCS Books.

Kreiß, C. (2015). *Gekaufte Forschung: Wissenschaft im Dienst der Konzerne* [Bought research: Science in the service of corporations]. Berlin: Europa Verlag.

Krimsky, S. (2003). *Science in the Private Interest: Has the Lure of Profits Corrupted Biomedical Research?* Lanham, Md.: Rowman & Littlefield.

Krimsky, S. (2019). *Conflicts of Interest in Science: How Corporate-Funded Academic Research Can Threaten Public Health*. New York: Hot Books.

Kuhn, T.S. (1962). *The Structure of Scientific Revolutions*. Chicago: Chicago University Press.

Last, W. (2008). Are most diseases caused by the medical system? *Nexus* magazine, 15 (2) Feb–March, available online at http://whale.to/a/last1.html.

Legge, D. (2019). Review essay: Capitalism, imperialism and class: essential foundations for a critical public health. *Critical Public Health*, 29 (5), pp. 624–31; available at https://tinyurl.com/5n985rf7.

Lester, D. & Parker, D. (2019). *What Really Makes You Ill? Why Everything You Thought You Knew About Disease Is Wrong*, ISBN-13: 978-1673104035.

Lester, D. & Parker, D. (2023). Is medical intervention the leading cause of death? *The Light* newspaper, 31, p. 20.

Lewis, D.L. (2014). *Science for Sale: How the US Government Uses Powerful Corporations and Leading Universities to Support Government Policies, Silence Top Scientists, Jeopardize Our Health, and Protect Corporate Profits*. New York: Skyhorse Publishing.

Lexchin, J. (1984). *The Real Pushers: A Critical Analysis of the Canadian Drug Industry*. Vancouver, BC: New Star Books.

Lexchin, J. (2018). The pharmaceutical industry in contemporary capitalism, *Monthly Review*, 69 (10), pp. 37–50.

McCartney, M. (2013). *The Patient Paradox: Why Sexed-up Medicine Is Bad for Your Health*. London: Pinter & Martin.

McGarity, T.D. & Wagner, W.E. (2008). *Bending Science: How Special Interests Corrupt Public Health Research*. Cambridge, Mass.: Harvard University Press.

Maio, G. (2014). *Geschäftsmodell Gesundheit – wie der Markt die Heilkunst abschafft* [Business model health: how the market is abolishing the art of healing]. Berlin: Suhrkamp Verlag AG.

Mann, H. (2009). Beware of polypharmacy in the elderly, *BMJ* (Mar. 8). Online at www.bmj.com/cgi/eletters/338/mar03_2/b873.

Masters, R. (2022a). *Rudolf Steiner and Social Reform: Three-folding and other Proposals*. Forest Row, East Sussex: Rudolf Steiner Press.

Masters, R. (2022b). Creating foundations for trust in public life – a threefold approach. *The Light* newspaper, 22, p. 12.

Masters, Richard (2023). Personal communication, 13 March.

Michaels, D. (2008). *Doubt Is Their Product: How Industry's Assault on Science Threatens Your Health*. Oxford: Oxford University Press.

Misselbrook, D. (2001). *Thinking about Patients*. Newbury, Berks: Petroc Press.

Moynihan, R. & Cassels, A. (2005). *Selling Sickness: How the World's Biggest Pharmaceutical Companies Are Turning Us All into Patients*. New York: Avalon.

Navarro, V. (1976). *Medicine under Capitalism*. London: Croom Helm.

Navarro, V. & Berman, D. (1983). *Health and Work under Capitalism: An International Perspective*. London: Routledge.

Null, G. (2011). *Death by Medicine*. Edinburgh, VA: Praktikos Books.

O'Mahony, S. (2019). *Can Medicine Be Cured? The Corruption of a Profession*. London: Head of Zeus / Apollo.

Patashnik, E.M., Gerber, A.S. & Dowling, C.M. (2017). *Unhealthy Politics: The Battle over Evidence-based Medicine*. Princeton, NJ: Princeton University Press.

Paulitz, H. (2016). *Anleitung gegen den Krieg – Analysen und friedenspolitische Übungen* [Manual against war – analyses and peace policy exercises]. Hamburg: Akademie Bergstraße.

Payer, L. (1992). *Disease-Mongers: How Doctors, Drug Companies, and Insurers are Making You Feel Sick*. New York: John Wiley.

Piketty, T. (2014). *Das Kapital im 21. Jahrhundert* [Capital in the 21st Century]. München: C.H. Beck.

Reiser, S.J. (1978). *Medicine and the Reign of Technology*. Cambridge: Cambridge University Press.

Ryder, R. (2021). *Medical Fascism: How Coronavirus Policy Took Our Freedoms way and How to Get Them Back*. ISBN 9798514158577.

Sharpe, V.A. & Faden, A.I. (1998). *Medical Harm: Historical, Conceptual and Ethical Dimensions of Iatrogenic Illness*. Cambridge: Cambridge University Press.

Sidhwa, K. (1976). *Medical Drugs on Trial? Verdict, 'Guilty!': An Exposé of the Present Day Practice of Medicine, the Drug Industry, and Food Technology*. Chicago: Natural Hygiene Press.

Sikorski, W. (2011). *Infected with Difference: Healing Dis/ease in the Body Politic*. CreateSpace Independent Publishing Platform.

Smith, W.J. (2016). *Culture of Death: The Age of 'Do Harm' Medicine*. New York: Encounter Books.

Sobel, D.S. (ed.) (1979). *Ways of Health: Holistic Approaches to Ancient and Contemporary Medicine*. New York: Harcourt Brace Jovanovich.

Stegenga, J. (2018). *Medical Nihilism*. Oxford: Oxford University Press.

Steiner, R. (2013). *Understanding Healing: Meditative Reflections on Deepening Medicine through Spiritual Science: 316* (Collected Works of Rudolf Steiner). Forest Row, East Sussex: Rudolf Steiner Press.

Taylor, R. (1979). *Medicine out of Control: The Anatomy of a Malignant Technology*. Melbourne: Sun Books.

Waitzkin, H. & others (2018). *Health Care under the Knife: Moving beyond Capitalism for our Health*. New York:

Monthly Review Press.

Walker, M.J. (1993). *Dirty Medicine: Science, Big Business and the Assault on Natural Health Care*. London: Slingshot Publications.

Walker, M.J. (2011). *Dirty Medicine Handbook*. London: Slingshot Publications.

Walker, M.J. (ed.) (2017). *Corporate Ties that Bind: An Examination of Corporate Manipulation and Vested Interest in Public Health*. New York: Skyhorse.

Weiss, H. (2007). *Bittere Pillen – Nutzen und Risiken der Arzneimittel* [Bitter pills: the uses and risks of medications]. Kiepenheuer & Witsch

Welch, H.G., Schwartz, L.M. & Woloshin, S. (2011). *Overdiagnosed: Making People Sick in the Pursuit of Health*. Boston, Mass.: Beacon Press.

Wilkinson, R. & Pickett, K. (2010). *The Spirit Level: Why Equality is Better for Everyone*. London: Penguin.

Ziegler, J. (2012). *Wir lassen sie verhungern – die Massenvernichtung in der dritten Welt* [We let them starve – the mass destruction in the third world]. München: C. Bertelsmann Verlag.

List of sources for figures

1. https://www.pinterest.de/artaud19/sascha-schneider/
2. Grafik: Helmut Creutz, from the book *Das Geld-Syndrom*, new edition 2012, from http://friedensblick.de/2017/jetzt-erfuellen-sich-ur-alte-warnungen-vor-dem-zins-mal-wieder/
3. https://www.gold.de/staatsverschuldung-deutschland/
4. https://tinyurl.com/4y4mefxp
5. http://www.sozialpolitik-aktuell.de/gesundheit-datensammlung.html
6. https://tinyurl.com/4a7hpknt
7. http://www.sozialpolitik-aktuell.de/einkommen-datensammlung.html
8. https://tinyurl.com/2rszbdtt (a page on handelsblatt.com). Figures on Rate of Return have been added, based on figures from http://www.boerse.de/performance/ , last accessed 2017.
9. Compiled by the author, Figures from Lit. 4
10. Süddeutsche Zeitung 18.3.2008, https://tinyurl.com/yzwzxzta
11. Süddeutsche Zeitung 10.4.2014, https://tinyurl.com/ycc2k65j
12. Put together by the author
13. Zeit online, https://tinyurl.com/5n6tw84j
14. https://de.wikipedia.org/wiki/Arbeitslosenstatistik
15. Wikipedia. https://tinyurl.com/44475v7f
16. – 25. From Wilkinson & Pickett, 2010 (see references)
26. Data from OECD, Health expenditures

About the authors

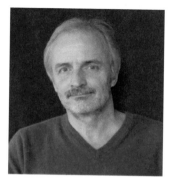

THOMAS HARDTMUTH, MD, studied human medicine at the TU and LMU Munich between 1978 and 1985. He trained as a consultant surgeon at Heidenheim Hospital and as a thoracic surgeon at Ulm University Hospital, and between 1996 and 2016 was senior physician at Heidenheim Hospital. From 2011 to 2020, Thomas was Lecturer in Health Sciences, Epidemiology and Social Medicine at the Baden-Württemberg Cooperative State University. For many years he was involved in the working group 'Projects of Goethean Science' at the Carl Gustav Carus Institute in Öschelbronn and in the microbiology working group at the Goetheanum in Dornach/Switzerland.

Other main research interests are neurobiology, oncology, health economics and the autonomy principle in salutogenesis. His publications include: *Das verborgene Ich – Aspekte zum Verständnis der Krebskrankheit* (Amthorverlag, 2003); *Denkfehler – das Dilemma der Hirnforschung* (Amthorverlag, 2006); *In der Dämmerung des Lebendigen – Hintergründe zu Demenz, Depression und Krebs* (Amthorverlag, 2011); 'Mikrobiom und erweiterter Organismusbegriff' (in *Jahrbuch für Goetheanismus,* 2017); *Mikrobiom und Mensch – Die Bedeutung der Mikroorganismen und Viren in Medizin, Evolution und Ökologie. Wege zu einer systemischen Perspektive* (Salumed-Verlag, 2021); *What Covid-19 Must Teach Us: Meeting Viruses with Fear or Informed Common Sense* (InterActions, 2022); *Beyond Mainstream Medicine: Dialogue Towards a New Paradigm for Health* (InterActions, 2022, with Richard House).

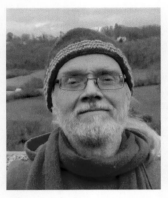

RICHARD HOUSE, MA [Oxon], Ph.D. is a chartered psychologist and freedom campaigner in Stroud, UK. Previously Senior Lecturer in Early Childhood, University of Winchester (2012–14) and Senior Lecturer in Psychotherapy and Psychology, University of Roehampton (2005–2012), Richard edits *Self and Society: International Journal for Humanistic Psychology*, and is a founding-member of the Independent Practitioners Network and the Alliance for Counselling & Psychotherapy. A trained Steiner kindergarten and class teacher, his several books on education include the acclaimed *Too Much, Too Soon? Early Learning and the Erosion of Childhood* (Hawthorn Press, 2011) and *Childhood, Well-being and a Therapeutic Ethos* (Karnac/Routledge 2009, with Del Loewenthal). A founding-member of the 'Open EYE' Campaign (openeyecampaign.wordpress.com/), Richard organised the three *Daily Telegraph* Open Letters on the state of modern childhood in 2006, 2007 (both with Sue Palmer) and in 2011. A former counsellor/psychotherapist and supervisor in general medical and private practice, he has published hundreds of articles, academic papers, book reviews and book chapters on a range of subjects (see tinyurl.com/2p8kmkyf and tinyurl.com/ydpw4u8x).

Research interests include the 'Audit Culture'; critical perspectives on technology and technocracy; discourses on the 'new world order'; and the work of Rudolf Steiner and Paul Feyerabend, with a particular current interest in contesting medical/healing paradigms.

Index

Additional titles by InterActions

See our website for further information – interactions360.org

Also by Thomas Hardtmuth (in English translation)

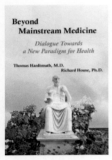

BEYOND MAINSTREAM MEDICINE: Dialogue towards a new paradigm for health

by Thomas Hardtmuth, MD and Richard House, PhD

2022. ISBN 978-0-9528364-8-3, Pb 150 pp, UK £11.99

This interview-dialogue dives deeply into the very foundations of human well-being, detailing what is wrong philosophically and clinically with the current biomedical paradigm of health and disease; how these shortcomings have been highlighted in the course of the Covid crisis; and what changes need to occur for the radical re-founding of a genuinely holistic understanding of health, illness and healing to occur.

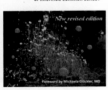

WHAT COVID-19 MUST TEACH US Meeting viruses with fear or informed common sense?

by Thomas Hardtmuth, MD
Foreword by Michaela Glöckler, MD

2nd edition, 2022. ISBN 978-0-9528364-7-6, Pb 122 pp, £8.95

Dr Hardtmuth provides a detailed and updated analysis of the multi-dimensional Corona crisis, with valuable insights relevant for any future health crisis. This includes an in-depth description of our immune system resilience; the latest science recognising viruses not as 'enemies' but as vital for human evolution and health; the use of PCR tests; risks of vaccinations during an epidemic; the significant impact of fear and negative publicity on immunity; and, importantly, the unhealthy relationship between politics, business and medicine.

Titles by other authors

BEING HUMAN IN THE NOW:
Conversations with the soul of my sister Ajra

by Ana Pogacnik

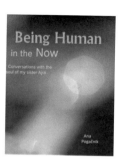

2022. ISBN 978-9528364-6-9, Pb 120 pp with illustrations, UK £12

Ten years after her death, the author takes up conversations with the soul of her departed sister, revealing profound insights into challenges humanity is facing. The themes covered are direct, detailed and breathtakingly lively and highly topical. Inspiring are the descriptions of the deep significance of love as a source of strength, and of the spiritually radiating living being we know as earth which we can learn to interact with. In all of this the message is: the departed souls are eager to work more closely with us, bringing healing and fertilisation for the present and future.

CORONA AND THE HUMAN HEART:
Illuminating riddles of immunity, conscience and common sense

by Michaela Glöckler, MD
Foreword by Branko Furst, MD

2021. ISBN 978-0-9528364-5-2, Pb 96 pp, UK £7.95
Colour and B&W illustrations

New inspiring research on the significant role of the heart in the development of the immune system and the importance this understanding has for any health crisis, whether Covid, Monkeypox or others. The author leads us on a path showing how, by strengthening our inner spiritual self — our inner sun — we will be strengthening our health and immunity, as well as illuminating riddles of conscience and common sense.

"This timely book represents a breakthrough in phenomenological research that will provide far-reaching insights..." B. Furst, M.D.

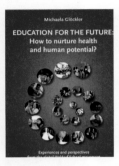

EDUCATION FOR THE FUTURE:
How to nurture health and human potential?

by Michaela Glöckler, MD

2020. ISBN 978-0-9528364-3-8, Pb 248 pp, UK £19.99, colour photos and illustrations

'Almost every day you can read somewhere that a fundamental change is needed in schools and the education system…' M.G.

Education for the Future is a plea for radically aligning upbringing and education with what is needed for the healthy development and well-being of children and adolescents. A unique contribution of Dr Glöckler is a year-by-year examination of human biological development and how this relates to soul-spiritual development, which in turn has a direct bearing on the needs of the child and what we can bring in the home and in education. It is the best prerequisite for a creative life into old age. A treasure chest of information and insights for educators, parents, carers and therapists alike.

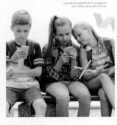

GROWING UP HEALTHY IN A WORLD OF DIGITAL MEDIA

A guide for parents and caregivers of children and adolescents

Written by specialists from 15 organisations concerned with media and childhood development. Introduction by Dr Michaela Glöckler.

2019. ISBN 9780 9528364 14, Pb 160 pp, UK £10, sewn binding, colour illustrations and photos.

With increased screen use following Covid epidemic restrictions, this new guide is more relevant than ever. It explains child development considerations, noting dangers of inappropriate use and giving practical advice for a positive *age appropriate* use of digital media. It integrates a holistic approach, with consideration of physical, emotional and mental development of children. Easy to read. *An essential guide.*

PUSHING BACK TO OFSTED

Safeguarding and the legitimacy of Ofsted's inspection judgements – a critical case study

by Richard House, PhD
Foreword by Prof. Saville Kushner.
2020, ISBN 978-0-9528364-2-1, Pb 128 pp,
UK £10.99

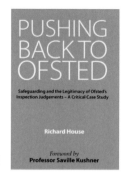

'Ofsted' (Office for Standards in Education) in England is considered to be one of the harshest school inspectorates in the world. Dr House wrote this book following the closure of several Waldorf schools in the UK due to Ofsted inspections. He sets out in relentless detail the shortcomings and prejudices of the Ofsted report for one of those schools, as an example for how a state's one-size-fits-all approach can perpetuate a kind of violence on educational creativity and freedoms. It is a helpful study for any school facing intense state scrutiny and judgement.

"There are crucial questions to answer about the fairness and effectiveness of an inspection culture that ignores or undermines the professional vision of teachers in their own schools. This analysis ... is an uncomfortable but necessary challenge to current educational orthodoxies."

Dr Rowan Williams, former Archbishop of Canterbury.

"This book ought to be read far and wide; being well informed will help us all in the time to come."

Dr James Dyson, Psychosynthesis Psychologist,
Physician, Co-founder of Park Attwood Clinic, Worcestershire

"We've known for years that something is fundamentally awry with modern medicine: this thought-provoking book sheds much light on why this might be so, challenges taken-for-granted narratives about healthcare, and describes innovative initiatives spawning all over the world that are pioneering a better, post-pharmaceutical approach to human health and well-being. Essential reading."

Dr Christian Buckland, Chair,
United Kingdom Council for Psychotherapy

"The first half of the book will have you shaking your head in disbelief; the second half vigorously nodding in agreement. Thomas Hardtmuth M.D. accurately diagnoses the problems in our current healthcare system and, thankfully, offers us some cures. With this glorious new book we are inching ever closer to a radical reorientation of healthcare and healing."

Dr Leah Gray,
Medical Doctor and Founder of Empower. Heal. Nourish.

"An important book that exposes the corruption in orthodox medicine due to the malign influence of Big Pharma, but also suggests positive solutions for the way forward."

Simon Best, MA
editor of *Caduceus* magazine (www.caduceus.info)

"A Must-Read to understand how Big Pharma plunder and destroy our real health needs. Important help to move towards the real health and well-being system we must build."

Piers Corbyn, Astrophysicist,
Meteorologist, political activist and freedom campaigner